SpringerBriefs in Materials

For further volumes:
http://www.springer.com/series/10111

Hendra Hermawan

Biodegradable Metals

From Concept to Applications

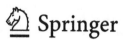 Springer

Hendra Hermawan
Faculty of Biomedical Engineering and Health Science
Universiti Teknologi Malaysia
Skudai 81310
Johor
Malaysia

ISSN 2192-1091   ISSN 2192-1105   (electronic)
ISBN 978-3-642-31169-7   ISBN 978-3-642-31170-3   (eBook)
DOI 10.1007/978-3-642-31170-3
Springer Heidelberg New York Dordrecht London

Library of Congress Control Number: 2012941639

Printed on acid-free paper

Springer is part of Springer Science+Business Media (www.springer.com)

Preface

Since their first introduction, metallic biomaterials have always been designed to be corrosion resistant. For decades, this paradigm has become the mainframe of the biomaterials world. It has been cited in thousands of scientific papers and taught in hundreds of courses of materials for biomedical devices. It has also been followed by industries in developing millions of medical devices until today.

Nowadays, with the advent of tissue engineering, biomaterials are envisaged to actively interact with the body. Metallic biomaterials are no more required to be inert but they should be able to assist and promote the healing process. In many cases, they should do their job and step away thereafter. This idea opens an extreme new horizon and provides new insight. One can imagine designing a material which is able to provide mechanical support for a required time and then progressively degrade. This idea directly breaks the paradigm of corrosion-resistant biomaterials.

Hundreds of publications on biodegradable metals are scattered in many journals since the first one published in 2001. Three consecutive annual international symposiums devoted to this emerging field have been held in Berlin (2009), Maratea (2010), and Quebec City (2011). Papers presented in those symposiums were published in special issues in Acta Biomaterialia (2010) and Materials Science and Engineering B (2011). This book, Biodegradable Metals: From Concept to Applications, should be the first to organize the scientific values of biodegradable metals research since the first decade of its development.

This book contains two main parts, each consisting of three chapters. The first part introduces the readers to the field of metallic biomaterials, exposes the state of the art of biodegradable metals, and reveals its application for cardiovascular implants. They were mostly compiled from the following publications: Hermawan et al. (2009a, 2010a, 2010b, 2011). The second part exposes an example of biodegradable metals from its concept to applications where a complete study on metallic biodegradable stent is detailed from materials design, development, testing till the implant fabrication. The second part was mostly compiled from my previous works on Fe-based alloys for biodegradable stents, mainly from my doctoral thesis submitted to Laval University in 2009, entitled: 'Conception, développement et validation d'alliages métalliques dégradables utilisés en chirurgie endovasculaire', with updates and benchmarking with recent similar works from other authors up to 2012.

I would like to sincerely thank my mentors, Prof. Diego Mantovani and Prof. Dominique Dube of Laval University, for their excellent supervision in my journey in developing expertise in biodegradable metals. I acknowledge the kindness of Dr. Lluis Duocastella of Iberhospitex Spain for giving me valuable experience in the stent fabrication process. I thank Dr. M. Rafiq of MediTeg Universiti Teknologi Malaysia and Mrs. Wang Dan of Biosensors Interventional Singapore for providing images of medical implants. I thank Dr. Yossi Febriani, Amelie and Maika for sacrificing their time during the completion of this book.

Bandung, June 2012   H. Hermawan

References

Hermawan, et al. (2009) Degradable metallic biomaterials: The concept, current developments and future directions, Minerva Biotecnologica 21:207–216

Hermawan, et al. (2010a) Degradable metallic biomaterials for cardiovascular applications, in Metals for Biomedical Devices, Woodhead Pub, Cambridge, pp 379–404

Hermawan, et al. (2010b) Developments in metallic biodegradable stents, Acta Biomaterialia 6:1693–1697

Hermawan, et al. (2011) Metals for biomedical applications, in Biomedical Engineering: from Theory to Applications, InTech Pub, Rijeka, pp 411–430

Contents

Chapter 1
Introduction to Metallic Biomaterials

Abstract After the invention of stainless steel in 1920s, metal implants have experienced vast development and clinical uses. The formation of ASTM Committee F04 on Medical and Surgical Materials and Devices in 1962 has then played important role to their development, practice and standardization. A great variety of corrosion resistant metals have been developed and used for medical implants including the class of 316L stainless steels, cobalt-chromium alloys and titanium and its alloys. New generation of metallic biomaterials have been made nickel free via novel processing including nano-processing and amorphization. Other development raised the concept of biodegradable rather than inert metals where temporary medical implants, that function only during specific period and then degrade, are targeted.

Keywords Biomaterial · Implant · Metal · Alloy

1.1 Brief Overview

The introduction of metal plate for bone fracture fixation by Lane more than a 100 years ago has marked the modern use of metals as medical implants (Lane 1895). Metals were chosen for use in the intervention of trauma, disease or malfunction of organs where loading present. In the early development, insufficient strength and corrosion were two main problems faced by metal implants (Lambotte 1909; Sherman 1912). In 1920s corrosion resistant 18-8 stainless steel was introduced and solved most of corrosion problem and thereafter fostered the vast development and clinical use of metal implants. In 1962 The American Society for Testing and Materials (ASTM) has formed Committee F04 on Medical and Surgical Materials and Devices to standardize metals for medical applications.

H. Hermawan, *Biodegradable Metals*, SpringerBriefs in Materials,
DOI: 10.1007/978-3-642-31170-3_1, © The Author(s) 2012

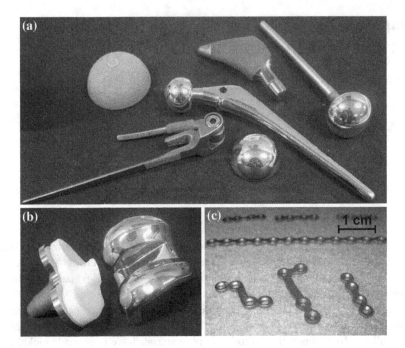

Fig. 1.1 Example of metallic implants for: **a** hip and elbow, **b** knee, **c** craniofacial. Courtesy of MediTeg, Universiti Teknologi Malaysia

Since then, the Committee has played a prominent role in all important aspects to materials, testing, devices and medical/surgical instruments.

Nowadays, hundreds of type of metals for implants has been used but in general they can be grouped into: (1) stainless steel alloys; (2) Co-Cr alloys; (3) Ti and its alloys; and (4) precious alloys. Figure 1.1 shows some examples of medical implants where metals are used.

The structural function and the inertness are two key features that make metallic biomaterials are in used. However, nowadays it is desirable that an implant also possesses bioactivities or biofunctionalities like blood compatibility and bone conductivity. Therefore surface modifications are required, i.e. to provide bone conductivity metal has been coated with hydroxyapatite (Habibovic et al. 2002), or with biopolymers to improve blood compatibility (Lahann et al. 1999). Today, development on metallic biomaterials includes those composed of nontoxic and allergy-free elements (Yang and Ren 2010) and biodegradable metals targeted for use as temporary implants (Hermawan and Mantovani 2009).

Table 1.1 Body environments to which metal implants are subjected

Condition	Parameters	Consequences
Body temperature	37 °C	Chemical reaction works faster than in ambient temperature
pH (Schneck 2000):		Even though body fluids are buffered solutions, pH temporary can decrease to ~5.2 around implantation site (Hench and Ethridge 1975).
• Blood	7.15–7.35	
• Intercellular matrix	7.0	
• Cells	6.8	
Dissolved oxygen (Black 1984):		Corrosive environment
• Arterial blood	100 mmHg	
• Venous blood	40 mmHg	
• Intercellular matrix	2–40 mmHg	
Chloride ion (Schneck 2000):		Corrosive environment
• Serum	113 mEq/l	
• Interstitial fluid	117 mEq/l	
Mechanical load (Niinomi 2010):		Could lead to fracture, stress corrosion cracking
• Cancellous bone	0–4 MPa	
• Cortical bone	0–40 MPa	
• Arterial wall	0.2–1 MPa	
• Myocardium	0–0.02 MPa	
• Muscle (max)	40 MPa	
• Tendon (max)	400 MPa	
Load repetition (Niinomi 2010):		Could lead to fatigue, wear and fretting
• Myocardial contraction	5×10^6– 4×10^7/ year	
• Finger joint exercise	10^5–10^6/year	
• Ambulation	2×10^6/year	

1.2 General Requirements

Metal implants are subjected to the conditions as described in Table 1.1. They are used in contact with living tissues thus they need to be biocompatible. Other functional characteristics that are important for metallic device include adequate mechanical properties such as strength, stiffness, and fatigue properties; and also appropriate density.

Metal implants are also required to be non-magnetic and have high density in order to be compatible with magnetic resonance imaging (MRI) techniques and to be visible under X-ray imaging. Most of artificial implants are subjected to loads,

Table 1.2 Implants division and type of metals used

Division	Implants	Type of metal
Orthopaedic	• Bone fixation (plate, screw, pin)	SS316L; Ti; Ti-6Al-4V
	• Spinal fixation	SS316L; Ti; Ti-6Al-4V; Ti-6Al-7Nb
	• Artificial joints	Co-Cr-Mo; T-6Al-4V; Ti-6Al-7Nb
Craniofacial	Plate and screw	SS316L; Co-Cr-Mo; Ti; Ti-6Al-4V
Cardiovascular	• Artificial valve	Ti-6Al-4V
	• Stent	SS316L; Co-Cr-Mo; Ti
	• Pace maker case	Ti; Ti-6Al-4V
	• Stent graft	SS316L
Otorhinology	• Artificial eardrum	SS316L
	• Artificial inner ear (electrode)	Pt
Dentistry	• Filling	Ag-Sn(-Cu) amalgam, Au
	• Inlay, crown, bridge	Au-Cu-Ag; Au-Cu-Ag-Pt-Pd; Ti; Co-Cr
	• Orthodontic wire	SS316L; Co-Cr-Mo; Ti-Ni; Ti-Mo
	• Dental implant	Ti; Ti-6Al-4V; Ti-6Al-7Nb; Au

either static or repetitive, and this condition requires an excellent combination of strength and ductility. This is the superiority of metals over polymers and ceramics.

Specific requirements of metals depend on the specific implant applications. Stents and stent grafts are implanted to open stenotic blood vessels; therefore, they require plasticity for expansion and rigidity for maintaining dilatation. In orthopaedic implant applications, metals are required to have excellent toughness, elasticity, rigidity, strength and resistance to fracture. Additionally, for total joint replacement metals are needed to be wear resistance to avoid debris formation from friction. Dental restoration requires strong and rigid metals and even the shape memory effect for better results.

1.3 Type of Mostly Used Metals

Type of metal used in biomedical depends on specific implant applications. The 316L type stainless steel (SS316L) is still the most used alloys in all implant division ranging from orthopaedic to dentistry. However, when an implant requires high wear resistance such as an artificial joint, Co-Cr alloys serve better. Table 1.2 summarized type of metals generally used for different implants division.

One of the basic characteristics of metals is their chemical composition which determines the formed microstructure and phases, thus their properties, i.e. mechanical properties. For example, the addition of Al and V into pure Ti greatly increase its tensile strength. Beside composition, metallurgical state of the metals changes their mechanical properties, i.e. annealed condition has better ductility than that of cold worked. The process to synthesis metals also affects their microstructure and properties. As an example, cast metal implants usually possess lower strength than those made by forging.

1.3.1 Stainless Steels

Up to now, the three most used metals for implants are stainless steel, Co-Cr alloys and Ti alloys. The first stainless steel used for implants contained $\sim 18wt\%$ Cr and $\sim 8wt\%$ Ni made it more resistant to corrosion and stronger than steel. The addition of Mo further improves its corrosion resistance, known as type 316 stainless steel. Further advancement was the reduction of its C content from 0.08 to 0.03wt% that improves corrosion resistance to Cl solution, and named as 316L. The ASTM has standardized stainless steel for surgical implants in their F138 (ASTM 2003), F899 (ASTM 2011a) and F2181 (ASTM 2009) standards.

1.3.2 Co-Cr Alloys

Co-Cr alloys are generally known for their excellent wear resistance where they have been in use in dentistry for many decades and in making artificial joints. Wrought Co-Ni-Cr-Mo alloy, for example, has been used for making loaded joints such as the hip and knee. ASTM standards covered these alloys include F75 (ASTM 2007a), F90 (ASTM 2007b), F562 (ASTM 2007c), F1537 (ASTM 2011b).

1.3.3 Ti and Ti Alloys

Having density only 4.5 g/cm^3, Ti is featured by its light weight compared to 7.9 g/cm^3 for 316 stainless steel and 8.3 g/cm^3 for cast Co-Cr-Mo alloys (Brandes and Brook 1992). The most known Ti alloys, Ti-6Al-4V, are considered as having excellent tensile strength and pitting corrosion resistance. When alloyed with Ni, Ti-Ni alloy or better known as Nitinol, possesses shape memory effect which is an interesting property used for example in dental restoration wiring. Titanium and its alloys for medical applications were covered in ASTM standards F67 (ASTM 2006), F136 (ASTM 2008) and F2063 (ASTM 2005).

1.3.4 Precious Alloys

Precious metals and alloys such as Au, Ag, Pt and their alloys are mostly known in dentistry due to their good castability, ductility and resistance to corrosion. Included into dental alloys are Au-Ag-Cu system, Au-Ag-Cu with the addition of Zn and Sn known as dental solder, and Au-Pt-Pd system used for porcelain-fused-to-metal for teeth repairs (John 2000).

Table 1.3 Materials commonly used for biomedical applications

Materials	Advantages	Disadvantages	Applications
Metals: stainless steel, Ti alloys, Co-Cr alloys, Mg alloys, etc.	Though, strong, ductile	Non bioactive	Load bearing implants; dental implants, joint replacement, cardiovascular stents, etc.
Ceramics: zirconia, alumina, bioglass, calcium phosphate, etc.	Bioactive, inert,	Brittle, not resilient	Orthopaedic and dental implants
Polymers: nylon, polylactide, polyethylene, polyesters, etc.	Bioactive, resilient	Not strong	Blood vessel grafts, sutures, hip sockets, etc.
Composites: amalgam, fiber-reinforced bone cement, etc.	Tailor made	Relatively difficult to make	Bone cement, dental resin

1.3.5 Other Metals and Alloys

Tantalum, amorphous alloys and biodegradable metals are among other metals used for implants. Due to its excellent X-ray visibility and low magnetic susceptibility, Ta is often used for X-ray markers for stents. Interesting properties have been shown by amorphous alloys compared to its crystalline counterparts whereas they exhibit a higher corrosion resistance, wear resistance, tensile strength and fatigue strength. Amorphous alloys like that of Zr-based (Wang et al. 2011) with its low Young's modulus may miniaturized metal implants. Amorphous Mg-based alloys have also shown a favorable degradation behavior where hydrogen evolution was not observed (Zberg et al. 2009).

1.4 Other Biomaterials

By definition, biomaterial is a nonviable material used in a medical device which is intended to interact with biological systems (Williams 1987). Biomaterials are used to make devices to replace a part or a function of the body in a reliable, safe, physiologically acceptable and economic manner (Park and Lakes 2007). It covers a broad range of materials from metals, ceramics and polymers, to composites. Table 1.3 summarizes materials commonly used as biomaterials.

1.4.1 Polymers

The main advantage of polymeric biomaterials over metals and ceramics is the ease of manufacturability to produce various shapes. Polymeric biomaterials can be divided into: (1) non-absorbable such as poly(methyl methacrylate), polyamide or nylon, poly(ethylene), etc.; and (2) absorbable such as poly(glycolide acid) and poly(lactide acid), etc. They can be a bulk or coating onto metal surfaces with tailored mechanical and physical properties. In recent development, absorbable polymers have been used for drug delivery carriers loaded with a specific drug in the form of coating on for example drug eluting stents. Jenkins has published a book which can be referred for further details on biomedical polymers (Jenkins 2007).

1.4.2 Ceramics

Ceramics biomaterials can be divided into: (1) inert bioceramics: zirconia, alumina, aluminum nitrides and carbon; (2) bioactive ceramics: hydroxyapatite, bioglass, etc.; (3) biodegradable/resorbable ceramics: calcium aluminates, calcium phosphates, etc. The inertness, high compressive strength and good appearance make ceramics attractive for dental crowns. Carbon has been used for heart valves exploiting its high specific strength and blood compatibility. Many bioceramics have been also applied as coating onto metal surfaces including nitrides, diamond like, carbon and more recently bioglasses and hydroxyapatites. A book written by Kokubo can be consulted for further reference on bioceramics (Kokubo 2008).

1.4.3 Composites

One example of composite biomaterial is bone. It is a composite of the low elastic modulus organic matrix reinforced with the high elastic modulus mineral "fibers" permeated with pores filled with liquids. Composites allow a control over material properties whereas a combination of stiff, strong, resilient but lightweight can be achieved all together. Other examples of biomedical composites include: orthopaedic implants with porous structures, dental filler, and bone cement composed of reinforced poly(methyl methacrylate) and ultra-high-molecular-weight poly(ethylene). Further reading on biomedical composites can be found in a book authored by Ambrosio (2009).

   Finally, biomaterials to be used clinically must be approved by authoritative bodies such as the United States Food and Drug Administration (FDA) or European conformity (CE) marking. The proposed biomaterial will be either granted Premarket Approval (PMA) if substantially similar to one used before the 1976 FDA legislation, or has to go through a series of guided biocompatibility assessments.

1.5 Recent Development

1.5.1 Low Elastic Modulus Alloys

In the recent development metallic biomaterials are desired to exhibit low elastic modulus, increased wear resistance and workability. Elastic moduli of Ti-Nb systems such as Ti-29Nb-13Ta-4.6Zr (Kuroda et al. 1998) and Ti-35Nb-4Sn (Matsumoto et al. 2005) can go down to 50–60 GPa which are closer to that of cortical bone (10–30 GPa). Wear resistance of cast Co-Cr alloy has been improved by maximizing C content and addition of Zr and N where optimal precipitation hardening permits the formation of fine and distributed carbides and the suppression of σ-phase (Lee et al. 2008). Improved workability of wrought Co-Cr alloys has been achieved by adding N to suppress carbides and intermetallics (Chiba et al. 2009).

1.5.2 Nickel-Free Alloys

Elimination of all possibility of toxic effects from leaching, wear and corrosion has become a great concern. Stainless steels have been further developed to be Ni-free by replacing Ni with other alloying elements while maintaining the stability of austenitic phase, corrosion resistance, magnetism and workability. This has lead to the use of N creating Fe-Cr-N, Fe-Cr-Mo-N and Fe-Cr-Mn-Mo-N systems (Yang and Ren 2010). The achieved higher strength opens the possibility for reduction of implant sizes where limited anatomical space is often an issue, for example, coronary stents with finer meshes (Yang and Ren 2010).

1.5.3 Metallic Glasses

A novel class of metals, metallic glasses, currently attracts attention from biomaterialist (Schroers et al. 2009). Nickel-free Zr based bulk metallic glasses represent their interesting properties where tensile strength, low elastic modulus and corrosion resistance are superior to those of crystalline alloys (Chen et al. 2010). These metals have high resistance to crystallization during cooling that allow the formation of bulk amorphous alloys or bulk metallic glasses (Johnson 2002). These alloys exhibit unusual combinations of engineering properties such as very high specific strength, and elastic strain limit which some are interesting for biomedical use.

1.5.4 Porous Metals

Apart from dense metallic biomaterials, porous structured metals offer further reduction on elastic modulus to get closer to that of cortical bone. This structure can be fabricated through powder sintering, space holder methods, decomposition of foaming agents and rapid prototyping (Ryan et al. 2006). A combination of rapid prototyping with investment casting (Lopez-Heredia et al. 2008), or powder sintering (Ryan et al. 2008), or 3D fiber deposition (Li et al. 2007) and or selective laser melting (Hollander et al. 2006) are some of promising processes for the development of porous metal structure for biomedical implants. Solid free form fabrication, a mouldless manufacturing techniques or rapid prototyping, have been successfully used to fabricate complex scaffolds. These technologies allow the preparation of tissue-engineered constructs with a controlled spatial distribution of cells and growth factors, also controlled gradients of scaffold materials with a targeted microstructure (Hutmacher et al. 2004).

1.5.5 Biodegradable Metals

With recent development in biotechnology, new concept of bioactive biomaterials, rather than inert biomaterials, was raised. A positive interaction of implant with the physiological site is promoted. Some level of biological activity is needed in particular area, such as in tissue engineering, where direct interactions between biomaterials and tissue components are very essential. In particular cases, biomaterials are needed only temporary and are expected to support the healing process and to thereafter degrade. These degradable biomaterials may be defined as materials used for medical implants which allow the implants to degrade in human body environment (Hermawan and Mantovani 2009). Biodegradable/bioabsorbable polymers were the first investigated for use as biomaterials (Stack et al. 1988). Meanwhile, the idea of considering biodegradable metals to fabricate temporary implants required in some sort to break the paradigm where corrosion resistance has always constituted one of the main requirements for metallic biomaterials. Further details about biodegradable metals will be discussed in the coming chapters.

1.6 Conclusion

Owing to their excellent biocompatibility and biofunctionality, ceramics and polymers have replaced some metal implants. However, those require high strength, toughness and durability, are still made of metals. With additional biofunctionalities and revolutionary use of metal such as for biodegradable implants, metals will continue to be used as biomaterials in the future. The direction goes toward the combination of the mechanically superior metals and the excellent biocompatibility and biofunctionality of ceramics and polymers to obtain the most desirable clinical performance of the implants.

References

Ambrosio L (2009) Biomedical composites. Woodhead Publishing, Cambridge

ASTM (2003) ASTM F 138: Standard specification for wrought 18chromium-14nickel-2.5molybdenum stainless steel bar and wire for surgical implants (UNS S31673). ASTM International, West Conshohocken

ASTM (2005) ASTM F 2063: standard specification for wrought nickel-titanium shape memory alloys for medical devices and surgical implants. ASTM International, West Conshohocken

ASTM (2006) ASTM F 67: standard specification for unalloyed titanium, for surgical implant applications (UNS R50250, UNS R50400, UNS R50550, UNS R50700). ASTM International, West Conshohocken

ASTM (2007a) ASTM F 75: standard specification for cobalt-28 chromium-6 molybdenum alloy castings and casting alloy for surgical implants (UNS R30075). ASTM International, West Conshohocken

ASTM (2007b) ASTM F 90: standard specification for wrought cobalt-20chromium-15tungsten-10nickel alloy for surgical implant applications (UNS R30605). ASTM International, West Conshohocken

ASTM (2007c) ASTM F 562: standard specification for wrought 35cobalt-35nickel-20chromium-10molybdenum alloy for surgical implant applications (UNS R30035). ASTM International, West Conshohocken

ASTM (2008) ASTM F 136: standard specification for wrought titanium-6 aluminum-4 vanadium ELI (extra low interstitial) alloy for surgical implant applications (UNS R56401). ASTM International, West Conshohocken

ASTM (2009) ASTM F 2181: standard specification for wrought seamless stainless steel tubing for surgical implants. ASTM International, West Conshohocken

ASTM (2011a) ASTM F 899: standard specification for wrought stainless steels for surgical instruments. ASTM International, West Conshohocken

ASTM (2011b) ASTM F 1537: standard specification for wrought cobalt-28chromium-6molybdenum alloys for surgical implants (UNS R31537, UNS R31538, and UNS R31539). ASTM International, West Conshohocken

Black J (1984) Biological performance of materials. Plenum Press, New York

Brandes EA, Brook GB (1992) Smithells metals reference book, 7th edn. Butterworth-Heinemann, Oxford

Chen Q, Liu L, Zhang S-M (2010) The potential of Zr-based bulk metallic glasses as biomaterials. Front Mater Sci China 4:34–44

Chiba A, Lee S-H, Matsumoto H, Nakamura M (2009) Construction of processing map for biomedical Co-28Cr-6Mo-0.16N alloy by studying its hot deformation behavior using compression tests. Mater Sci Eng A 513–514:286–293

Habibovic P, Barrère F, Blitterswijk CAV, Groot Kd, Layrolle P (2002) Biomimetic hydroxyapatite coating on metal implants. J Am Ceram Soc 83:517–522

Hench LL, Ethridge EC (1975) Biomaterials: the interfacial problem. Adv Biomed Eng 5:35–150

Hermawan H, Mantovani D (2009) Degradable metallic biomaterials: the concept, current developments and future directions. Minerva Biotecnol 21:207–216

Hollander DA, von Walter M, Wirtz T, Sellei R, Schmidt-Rohlfing B, Paar O, Erli H-J (2006) Structural, mechanical and in vitro characterization of individually structured Ti-6Al-4V produced by direct laser forming. Biomaterials 27:955–963

Hutmacher DW, Sittinger M, Risbud MV (2004) Scaffold-based tissue engineering: rationale for computer-aided design and solid free-form fabrication systems. Trends Biotechnol 22:354–362

Jenkins M (2007) Biomedical polymers. Woodhead Publishing, Cambridge

John CW (2000) Biocompatibility of dental casting alloys: a review. J Pros Dent 83:223–234

Johnson W (2002) Bulk amorphous metal—an emerging engineering material. J Min Met Mat Soc 54:40–43

Kokubo T (2008) Bioceramics and their clinical applications. Woodhead Publishing, Cambridge

Kuroda D, Niinomi M, Morinaga M, Kato Y, Yashiro T (1998) Design and mechanical properties of new [beta] type titanium alloys for implant materials. Mater Sci Eng A 243:244–249

Lahann J, Klee D, Thelen H, Bienert H, Vorwerk D, Hocker H (1999) Improvement of haemocompatibility of metallic stents by polymer coating. J Mater Sci Mater Med 10:443–448

Lambotte A (1909) Technique et indication des prothèses dans le traitement des fractures. Presse Med 17:321

Lane WA (1895) Some remarks on the treatment of fractures. Brit Med J 1:861–863

Lee SH, Nomura N, Chiba A (2008) Significant improvement in mechanical properties of biomedical Co-Cr-Mo alloys with combination of N addition and Cr-enrichment. Mater Trans 49:260–264

Li JP, Habibovic P, van den Doel M, Wilson CE, de Wijn JR, van Blitterswijk CA, de Groot K (2007) Bone ingrowth in porous titanium implants produced by 3D fiber deposition. Biomaterials 28:2810–2820

Lopez-Heredia MA, Sohier J, Gaillard C, Quillard S, Dorget M, Layrolle P (2008) Rapid prototyped porous titanium coated with calcium phosphate as a scaffold for bone tissue engineering. Biomaterials 29:2608–2615

Matsumoto H, Watanabe S, Hanada S (2005) Beta TiNbSn alloys with low Young's modulus and high strength. Mater Trans 46:1070–1078

Niinomi M (2010) Metals for biomedical devices. Woodhead Publishing, Cambridge

Park JB, Lakes RS (2007) Biomaterials: an introduction, 3rd edn. Springer, New York

Ryan G, Pandit A, Apatsidis DP (2006) Fabrication methods of porous metals for use in orthopaedic applications. Biomaterials 27:2651–2670

Ryan GE, Pandit AS, Apatsidis DP (2008) Porous titanium scaffolds fabricated using a rapid prototyping and powder metallurgy technique. Biomaterials 29:3625–3635

Schneck DJ (2000) The biomedical engineering handbook. CRC Press LLC, Boca Raton

Schroers J, Kumar G, Hodges T, Chan S, Kyriakides T (2009) Bulk metallic glasses for biomedical applications. J Min Met Mater Soc 61:21–29

Sherman WO (1912) Vanadium steel bone plates and screws. Surg Gynecol Obstet 14:629–634

Stack RS, Califf RM, Phillips HR, Pryor DB, Quigley PJ, Bauman RP, Tcheng JE, Greenfield JC Jr (1988) Interventional cardiac catheterization at Duke Medical Center. Am J Cardiol 62:3F–24F

Wang YB, Zheng YF, Wei SC, Li M (2011) In vitro study on Zr-based bulk metallic glasses as potential biomaterials. J Biomed Mater Res B 96:34–46

Williams DF (ed) (1987) Definitions in biomaterials. In: Progress in biomedical engineering. Elsevier, Amsterdam

Yang K, Ren Y (2010) Nickel-free austenitic stainless steels for medical applications. Sci Technol Adv Mater 11:1–13

Zberg B, Uggowitzer PJ, Loffler JF (2009) MgZnCa glasses without clinically observable hydrogen evolution for biodegradable implants. Nat Mater 8:887–891

Chapter 2
Biodegradable Metals: State of the Art

Abstract Degradable biomaterials constitute a novel class of bioactive biomaterials which are expected to support healing process of a diseased tissue and to degrade thereafter. Two classes of metals have been proposed: magnesium- and iron-based alloys. Three targeted applications are envisaged: orthopaedic, cardiovascular and pediatric implants. Conceptually, biodegradable metals should provide a temporary support on healing process and should progressively degrade thereafter.

Keywords Biodegradable metals · Degradation · Temporary implant

2.1 Paradigm Shifted

The scientific knowledge about tissue-implant interactions, tissue engineering, as well as recent advances in biology and physiology raises a new concept of biofunctional/bioactive biomaterials. These unconventional bioactive biomaterials are expected to promote positive interactions with the physiological implantation sites. Degradable biomaterials constitute a novel class of considerably bioactive biomaterials which are expected to support healing process of a diseased tissue or organ and slowly degrading thereafter. The study of innovative degradable biomaterials is one of the most interesting research topics at the forefront of biomaterials in present days.

The advancement of materials science and engineering, especially for processing and thermomechanical treatments, allow the structural material adjustment to meet the expected properties of materials. The increasing society expectation for a better quality of life has fostered biomaterialists to develop new technologies to provide implants with higher clinical performance. The paradigm of implants must be inert and corrosion resistant has now been challenged by the advent of this new class of degradable biomaterials.

H. Hermawan, *Biodegradable Metals*, SpringerBriefs in Materials,
DOI: 10.1007/978-3-642-31170-3_2, © The Author(s) 2012

Some specific clinical problems (disease/trauma) need only temporary support for healing. This temporary support can only be provided by an implant made of degradable biomaterials which allow the implant to progressively degrade after fulfilling its function. The concept of biodegradation has been known in medical applications, such as the use of biodegradable sutures. However, implants that degrade, especially those made of metal, can be considered as a novel concept which actually breaks the established paradigm of "metallic biomaterials must be corrosion resistant".

Degradable biomaterials have been proposed from both polymers and metals. Degradable polymers for use as biomaterials have been investigated since 1988 (Stack et al. 1988). Among the polymers that have been proposed were poly(L-lactic acid) (PLLA) (Stack et al. 1988; Tamai et al. 2000), poly(lactic-co-glycolic acid) (PLGA) and poly(ε-caprolactone) (PCL) (van der Giessen et al. 1996).

Considering metals as degradable biomaterials is a recent idea. In term of mechanical property, metals are considered as more suitable compared to polymers for some specific applications which require high strength to bulk ratio, including for internal bone fixation screws/pins and for coronary stents.

Magnesium- and Fe-based alloys are the two classes of metals have been proposed. Several Mg-based alloys have been investigated, including Mg–Al—(Heublein et al. 2003; Levesque et al. 2003; Witte et al. 2005; Xin et al. 2007), Mg–RE (rare earth)—(Di Mario et al. 2004; Peeters et al. 2005; Witte et al. 2005; Waksman et al. 2006; Hänzi et al. 2009) and Mg–Ca—(Zhang and Yang 2008; Li et al. 2008) based alloys.

Among the Fe-based alloys have been studied, including pure Fe (Peuster et al. 2001; Peuster et al. 2006) and Fe–Mn alloys (Hermawan et al. 2008; Schinhammer et al. 2010). They were mainly proposed for cardiovascular applications.

2.2 The Concept

In general, the concept of degradable biomaterials is as simple as that, some implants might require only temporary presence for supporting the healing process of a diseased tissue. This temporary intervention (implant) is envisaged to be applied in some specific cases such as in cardiovascular, orthopaedic and paediatric field. Figure 2.1 illustrates an example of envisaged temporary implant (stent) which is implanted to open a narrowed artery.

Those envisaged temporary implants possess a similar concept but employed in different physiological environments with different specific functions. In example, temporary cardiovascular implants, i.e. stents (Fig. 2.1), should be able to open a narrowed artery and hold it open until the vessel remodels, and then they degrade and are replaced by new arterial vessel tissue. Temporary orthopaedic implants, i.e. bone fixation screws/pins, should be able to join a fractured bone and hold it tight until sufficient bone joint is formed and then degrade and are replaced by new

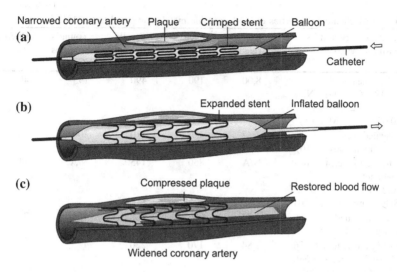

Fig. 2.1 Illustration of a coronary stent during it's: **a** delivery into a narrowed artery by a catheter, **b** expansion to open the artery, **c** restoring the blood flow. Adapted with permission from Minerva Medica (Hermawan and Mantovani 2009)

bone tissue. In paediatric, the implants should also deal with the growing implantation sites, the surrounding tissue and organ.

Ideally, biodegradable coronary stents should reach a compromise between mechanical integrity and degradation (Hermawan et al. 2010). The degradation should begin at a very slow rate to keep the stent's optimal mechanical integrity until the arterial vessel remodeling process completed which is expected in a period of 6–12 months (El-Omar et al. 2001; Schomig et al. 1994). Thereafter, while the mechanical integrity decreases, the degradation progresses. The degradation rate should be sufficient enough to do not cause an intolerable accumulation of degradation product around the implantation site and in the systemic organs. A reasonable total period for the stent to be totally degraded could be between 12 and 24 months after implantation (Serruys et al. 2006). However, this time frame is still not supported by sufficient data and evidences from the real degradation behavior in vivo, including that for orthopaedic implants.

In other words, the concept of biodegradable metals is *"providing a temporary support on healing process of a diseased tissue and progressively degrade thereafter"*. It derives two main features: (1) temporary support; and (2) degradation. Biodegradable metals are also expected to positively interact (bioactive) during the healing process. The metals, the degradation and its products are not supposed to provide adverse effect to the healing process.

Table 2.1 Mechanical properties of biodegradable metals compared to SS316L

Metal, metallurgy and its composition (wt%)	Density (g/cm^3)	Yield strength (MPa)	Tensile strength (MPa)	Young's modulus (GPa)	Ductility (%)
SS316L, annealed plate Fe, 16–18.5 Cr, 10–14 Ni, 2–3 Mo, <2 Mn, <1 Si, <0.03 C (ASTM 2003)[a]	8.00	190	490	193	40
Fe, annealed plate 99.8 Fe (Goodfellow 2010)	7.87	150	210	200	40
Fe-Mn-Pd alloy, cast + heat treatment Fe, 10.2 Mn, 0.92 Pd, 0.12 C (Schinhammer et al. 2010)	N/A	850	1450	N/A	11
Mg, annealed sheet 99.98 Mg (ASM 2005)	1.74	90	160	45	3
WE43 Mg alloy, temper T6 Mg, 3.7–4.3 Y, 2.4–4.4 Nd, 0.4–1 Zr (ASTM 2001)	1.84	170	220	44	2
Mg-Ca alloy, extruded Mg, 1 Ca (Li et al. 2008)	N/A	140	240	N/A	11

[a] Non-degradable, taken for comparison purpose. The values shown here are the minimum requirements by ASTM

2.3 Proof of Concept

2.3.1 Mechanical Support

The mechanical properties of metal are derived from its type, design and process. This includes the use of alloying elements, thermomechanical treatments and by employing new processing methods. The use of alloying elements which can form corrosion protective layer on the surface of materials; i.e. Cr for the case of stainless steel, should be avoided in order to ensure the alloys to become degradable or not corrosion resistant.

Biodegradable metals should provide an adequate mechanical support to a healing process throughout the implantation period. Even though it is still difficult to define the exact required support for specific clinical events, i.e. narrowed artery or fractured bone, it is reasonable to compare to the mechanical property of currently used corrosion-resistant metals. Table 2.1 resumes mechanical properties of Fe, Mg and their alloys compared to the known clinically proven metallic biomaterials, the SS316L.

Mechanical integrity of biodegradable metals over time can be theoretically predicted by conducting in vitro degradation tests. Kannan et al. have conducted a slow strain rate test on Mg-Al alloys allowing the measurement of mechanical properties as a function of degradation (Kannan and Raman 2008). The results showed that the elongation to fracture and ultimate tensile strength of AZ91Ca alloy in modified-simulated body fluid (SBF) decreased about 15–20 % in comparison with these properties in air.

2.3.2 Degradation

Biodegradable metals must degrade in the complex physiological environment of human body with matching degradation kinetics to the healing period. The degradation products should be transported and eliminated from the body and do not cause local or systemic accumulation. Table 2.2 summarizes published implantation studies of biodegradable metal intended for orthopaedic implants in animals. It briefly details the type of alloy and implant prototype, method of implantation; host, site, period and analysis, and some important findings.

The animal implantation studies showed that the proposed biodegradable metal implants were degraded under in vivo environment. In cardiovascular environment, generally the implants showed obvious sign of degradation in less than 1 month after implantation (Waksman et al. 2006, 2008). Magnesium alloy implants degrade faster than those of pure Fe, whereas Mg alloy stent completely degraded in less than 6 months (Waksman et al. 2006), meanwhile parts of pure Fe stents were still visible after a year of implantation (Peuster et al. 2001). In bone environment, Mg alloy pins degraded within 3 months and were replaced by new bone tissue (Li et al. 2008).

Absence of degradation products accumulation and signs of metal overload or metal-related organ toxicity (heart, lung, spleen, liver, kidney and para-aortic lymphatic nodes) were confirmed for Fe stents (Peuster et al. 2001, 2006). Examination of the blood has shown that the degradation of Mg implant caused only little change to the composition without disorder to liver or kidneys (Zhang et al. 2009). Similar finding showed no statistically significant differences of serum Mg before operation and at 1, 2, 3 months post-operation, suggesting the functionality of self-regulation mechanism of organism and excretion of surplus Mg from urine (Li et al. 2008).

2.4 Recent Development

Most of works on biodegradable metals covers materials development, property enhancement, degradation study and in vivo implantation of the material. There is still limited work that transformed biodegradable metals into implant or prototype. Among the developed implants are Fe-Mn alloy coronary stent (Hermawan and Mantovani 2011), WZ21 Mg alloy gastrointestinal would closure (Hänzi et al. 2011) and Mg micro-clip for laryngeal micro-surgery (Chng et al. 2012), (Fig. 2.2).

Table 2.2 Implantation of biodegradable metals in animal

Materials	Methods	Findings
Mg-Al/Y/Li/RE alloys pins (Witte et al. 2005)	Implantation on femora of 40 guinea pigs for a period up to 18 weeks, followed by radiography and histology	The corrosion layer of the rods displayed accumulation of biological Ca/P while in direct contact with the surrounding bone; subcutaneous gas bubbles formed after 1 week and disappear in 2–3 week but no adverse effect was observed
Mg-Ca alloy pins (Li et al. 2008)	Implantation on femora of: 18 New Zealand rabbits for a period up to 3 months, followed by radiography and histology	Gas bubbles formed in a week and disappear later without special treatment; the pins gradually degraded in vivo within 90 days; newly formed bone was clearly seen at month 3
Mg-Zn-Mn alloy rods (Zhang et al. 2009)	Implantation on femora of 18 rats for a period up to 26 weeks, followed by blood test and histology	No gas bubble was observed, new bone tissue formed around Mg implants after 6 weeks; higher degradation rate was found in the marrow channel than in the cortical bone tissue; little change to blood composition without disorder to liver or kidneys
Mg-0.8Ca screws (Erdmann et al. 2011)	Implantation on tibiae of 40 rabbits up to 8 weeks, followed by micro-CT and remnant analysis	The screws showed good tolerability and biomechanical properties comparable with S316L in the first 2–3 weeks post-implantation; They gradually degraded and became distinct after 6 weeks resulted in a loss of holding power; further investigation on the relation of the reduced holding power and bone healing was suggested especially with the combination of screw and plate
ZX50 and WZ21 alloys pin (Kraus et al. 2012)	Implantation on femora of 32 Sprague–Dawley rats up to 24 weeks, followed by online micro-CT monitoring and histology	ZX50 pins degraded at $\approx 1.2\%$ daily volume loss, WZ21 pins maintained their integrity for 4 weeks and degraded at $\sim 0.5\%$ volume loss per day; WZ21 generated enhanced bone neoformation with evidence for good osteoconductivity and osteoinductivity; bone recovered after complete degradation
Mg-Zn-Ca alloy rods (Chen et al. 2012)	Implantation on femur shaft of rabbits for a period up to 50 weeks, followed by radiography, micro-CT and histology	HA-composite coated rods degraded slower than the uncoated; the coated rods induced more newly formed bone tissue and faster bone response

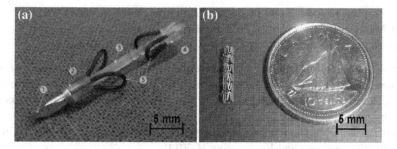

Fig. 2.2 Examples of implant prototype developed from biodegradable metals: **a** a wound closing rivet made of WZ21 Mg alloy, adapted with permission from Elsevier (Hänzi et al. 2011), **b** a coronary stent made of Fe-35Mn alloy, courtesy of Centre de recherche du CHUQ, Quebec, Canada

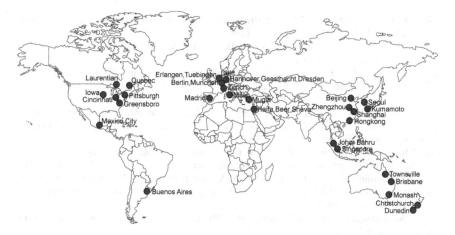

Fig. 2.3 Map of research groups working on biodegradable metals as of 2012

Up to now, proposed biodegradable metals can be identified as:

1. Mg-based alloys both conventionally produced through casting or by fine microstructure oriented processes;
2. Pure Fe and Fe-based alloys which were produced by casting, mechanical alloying or electrodeposition;
3. Metallic glasses which have been developed from both Mg- and Fe-based alloys.

The growing interest toward biodegradable metals was recorded in both journal database such as in the US National Library of Medicine and the National Institutes of Health (PubMed 2011) and in patent database such as the United States Patent and Trademark Office (USPTO 2011). Three consecutive international symposiums on biodegradable metals for biomedical applications were successfully held:

1. During the Thermec'2009 in Berlin, Germany, 25–29 August 2009;
2. In Maratea, Italy, 31 August-3 September 2010; and
3. During the Thermec'2011 in Quebec City, Canada, 1–5 August 2011.

It was revealed from those symposiums that the field has gained attentions from researchers around the world including from Canada, USA, Australia, Germany, Swiss, Japan, China, Mexico, and New Zealand. Figure 2.3 maps the groups working on biodegradable metals created based on their participation in the three symposiums and its publications in the special issues of Acta Biomaterialia 2010 and Materials Science and Engineering B 2011.

References

ASM (2005) ASM handbook, vol 2: Properties and selection: nonferrous alloys & special purpose materials. ASM International, Materials Park

ASTM (2001) ASTM B 80: standard specification for magnesium-alloy sand castings. ASTM International, West Conshohocken

ASTM (2003) ASTM F 138: standard specification for wrought 18chromium-14nickel-2.5molybdenum stainless steel bar and wire for surgical implants (UNS S31673). ASTM International, West Conshohocken

Chen S, Guan S, Li W, Wang H, Chen J, Wang Y (2012) In vivo degradation and bone response of a composite coating on Mg-Zn-Ca alloy prepared by microarc oxidation and electrochemical deposition. J Biomed Mater Res B 100:533–543

Chng CB, Lau DP, Choo JQ, Chui CK (2012) Bio-absorbable micro-clip for laryngeal microsurgery—design and evaluation. Acta Biomater. doi:10.1016/j.actbio.2012.1003.1051

Di Mario C, Griffiths H, Goktekin O, Peeters N, Verbist J, Bosiers M, Deloose K, Heublein B, Rohde R, Kasese V, Ilsley C, Erbel R (2004) Drug-eluting bioabsorbable magnesium stent. J Interv Cardiol 17:391–395

El-Omar MM, Dangas G, Iakovou I, Mehran R (2001) Update on in-stent restenosis. Curr Interv Cardiol Rep 3:296–305

Erdmann N, Angrisani N, Reifenrath J, Lucas A, Thorey F, Bormann D, Meyer-Lindenberg A (2011) Biomechanical testing and degradation analysis of MgCa0.8 alloy screws: a comparative in vivo study in rabbits. Acta Biomater 7:1421–1428

Goodfellow (2010) Iron (Fe)—material information (2010) Goodfellow Corp. http://www.goodfellow.com/csp/active/STATIC/A/Iron.HTML. Accessed 5 December 2010

Hänzi AC, Sologubenko AS, Uggowitzer PJ (2009) Design strategy for microalloyed ultra-ductile magnesium alloys for medical applications. Mater Sci Forum 618–619:75–82

Hänzi AC, Metlar A, Schinhammer M, Aguib H, Lüth TC, Löffler JF, Uggowitzer PJ (2011) Biodegradable wound-closing devices for gastrointestinal interventions: degradation performance of the magnesium tip. Mater Sci Eng C 31:1098–1103

Hermawan H, Mantovani D (2009) Degradable metallic biomaterials: the concept, current developments and future directions. Minerva Biotecnol 21:207–216

Hermawan H, Mantovani D (2011) New generation of medical implants: metallic biodegradable coronary stent. In: 2nd international conference on instrumentation, communications, information technology, and biomedical engineering (ICICI-BME), Bandung, 8–9 November 2011, pp 399–402

Hermawan H, Alamdari H, Mantovani D, Dubé D (2008) Iron-manganese: new class of degradable metallic biomaterials prepared by powder metallurgy. Powder Metall 51:38–45

Hermawan H, Dube D, Mantovani D (2010) Developments in metallic biodegradable stents. Acta Biomater 6:1693–1697

Heublein B, Rohde R, Kaese V, Niemeyer M, Hartung W, Haverich A (2003) Biocorrosion of magnesium alloys: a new principle in cardiovascular implant technology. Heart 89:651–656

Kannan MB, Raman RKS (2008) In vitro degradation and mechanical integrity of calcium-containing magnesium alloys in modified-simulated body fluid. Biomaterials 29:2306–2314

Kraus T, Fischerauer SF, Hänzi AC, Uggowitzer PJ, Löffler JF, Weinberg AM (2012) Magnesium alloys for temporary implants in osteosynthesis: in vivo studies of their degradation and interaction with bone. Acta Biomater 8:1230–1238

Levesque J, Dube D, Fiset M, Mantovani D (2003) Investigation of corrosion behaviour of magnesium alloy AM60B-F under pseudo-physiological conditions. Mater Sci Forum 426–432:521–526

Li Z, Gu X, Lou S, Zheng Y (2008) The development of binary Mg-Ca alloys for use as biodegradable materials within bones. Biomaterials 29:1329–1344

Peeters P, Bosiers M, Verbist J, Deloose K, Heublein B (2005) Preliminary results after application of absorbable metal stents in patients with critical limb ischemia. J Endovasc Ther 12:1–5

Peuster M, Wohlsein P, Brugmann M, Ehlerding M, Seidler K, Fink C, Brauer H, Fischer A, Hausdorf G (2001) A novel approach to temporary stenting: Degradable cardiovascular stents produced from corrodible metal-results 6–18 months after implantation into New Zealand white rabbits. Heart 86:563–569

Peuster M, Hesse C, Schloo T, Fink C, Beerbaum P, Schnakenburg CV (2006) Long term biocompatibility of a corrodible peripheral iron stent in the porcine descending aorta. Biomaterials 27:4955–4962

Schinhammer M, Hänzi AC, Löffler JF, Uggowitzer PJ (2010) Design strategy for biodegradable Fe-based alloys for medical applications. Acta Biomater 6:1705–1713

Schomig A, Kastrati A, Mudra H, Blasini R, Schuhlen H, Klauss V, Richardt G, Neumann FJ (1994) Four-year experience with Palmaz-Schatz stenting in coronary angioplasty complicated by dissection with threatened or present vessel closure. Circulation 90:2716–2724

Serruys PW, Kutryk MJ, Ong AT (2006) Coronary-artery stents. N Engl J Med 354:483–495

Stack RS, Califf RM, Phillips HR, Pryor DB, Quigley PJ, Bauman RP, Tcheng JE, Greenfield JC Jr (1988) Interventional cardiac catheterization at Duke Medical Center. Am J Cardiol 62:3F–24F

Tamai H, Igaki K, Kyo E, Kosuga K, Kawashima A, Matsui S, Komori H, Tsuji T, Motohara S, Uehata H (2000) Initial and 6-month results of biodegradable poly-l-lactic acid coronary stents in humans. Circulation 102:399–404

United States Patent and Trademark Office (2011). http://www.uspto.gov. Accessed 30 Oct 2011

US National Library of Medicine and the National Institutes of Health (2011). http://www.ncbi.nlm.nih.gov/pubmed. Accessed 30 Oct 2011

van der Giessen WJ, Lincoff AM, Schwartz RS, van Beusekom HM, Serruys PW, Holmes DR Jr, Ellis SG, Topol EJ (1996) Marked inflammatory sequelae to implantation of biodegradable and nonbiodegradable polymers in porcine coronary arteries. Circulation 94:1690–1697

Waksman R, Pakala R, Kuchulakanti PK, Baffour R, Hellinga D, Seabron R, Tio FO, Wittchow E, Hartwig S, Harder C, Rohde R, Heublein B, Andreae A, Waldmann K-H, Haverich A (2006) Safety and efficacy of bioabsorbable magnesium alloy stents in porcine coronary arteries. Catheter Cardiovasc Interv 68:606–617

Waksman R, Pakala R, Baffour R, Seabron R, Hellinga D, Tio FO (2008) Short-term effects of biocorrodible iron stents in porcine coronary arteries. J Interv Cardiol 21:15–20

Witte F, Kaese V, Haferkamp H, Switzer E, Linderberg AM, Wirth CJ, Windhagen H (2005) In vivo corrosion of four magnesium alloys and the associated bone response. Biomaterials 26:3557–3563

Xin Y, Liu C, Zhang X, Tang G, Tian X, Chu PK (2007) Corrosion behavior of biomedical AZ91 magnesium alloy in simulated body fluids. J Mater Res 22:2004–2011

Zhang E, Yang L (2008) Microstructure, mechanical properties and bio-corrosion properties of Mg-Zn-Mn-Ca alloy for biomedical application. Mater Sci Eng, A 497:111–118

Zhang E, Xu L, Yu G, Pan F, Yang K (2009) In vivo evaluation of biodegradable magnesium alloy bone implant in the first 6 months implantation. J Biomed Mater Res A 90:882–893

Chapter 3
Biodegradable Metals for Cardiovascular Applications

Abstract From basically pure magnesium and pure iron, the choice and technology for proposed biodegradable metals for cardiovascular applications have been progressed. These metals have been tested and validated by in vitro, in vivo till pre-clinical and clinical testing. Even though, lessons from their 10 years development indicated that the ideal characteristics of both the metals and the implants are yet to be achieved.

Keywords Cardiovascular · Stent · Biodegradable metal · Magnesium · Iron

3.1 The Need for Biodegradable Stent

Stenting, clinically known as percutaneous coronary intervention (PCI), has become a proven procedure for the treatment of coronary artery occlusions (Serruys et al. 2006). During stenting, one or more stent is delivered and placed into a narrowed coronary artery by using a catheter system that is inserted into the artery through a small incision in arm or groin (King et al. 2008). Stent provides a mechanical scaffolding support and prevent early recoil and late vascular remodeling, the two major limitations of balloon angioplasty (Serruys et al. 1994; Fischman et al. 1994). Figure 3.1 shows some examples of coronary stents which include corrosion resistant stents and metallic biodegradable stents.

Since its first introduction in 1987 (Sigwart et al. 1987), stenting and stent technology has progressively been advanced from the conventional bare metal stents to the drug eluting stents and the most recent biodegradable stents (Elliot et al. 2006; Waksman 2007; Hermawan et al. 2010). These tiny tubular mesh-like structures are currently made from corrosion resistant alloys, such as SS316L, Co–Cr alloys and Ni–Ti alloys. Typical diameter of large coronary artery is 2–5 mm with vessel thickness of 0.5–1 mm (Schneck 2000). Meanwhile, a stainless steel

H. Hermawan, *Biodegradable Metals*, SpringerBriefs in Materials,
DOI: 10.1007/978-3-642-31170-3_3, © The Author(s) 2012

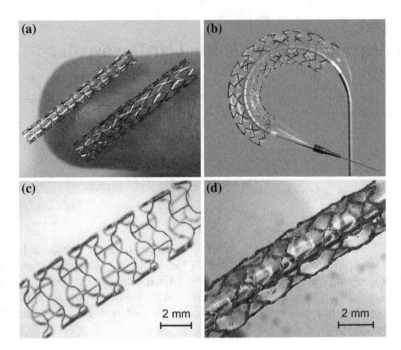

Fig. 3.1 Example of coronary artery stents: **a, b** inert type made of SS316L, courtesy of Biosensors International, Singapore, **c, d** biodegradable type made of Mg alloy and Fe, respectively, adapted with permission from Elsevier (Erbel et al. 2007) and Cambridge University Press (Peuster et al. 2006a), respectively

coronary stent for small vessel is typically produced at 1.8 mm external diameter, then crimped into balloon catheter at 1.05 mm and set for expansion at 3.0 mm. Pressure required to well positioned a stainless steel stent typically is 10–14 atm (1.0–1.4 MPa) (Colombo et al. 1995) which give a plastic deformation to the stent's strut up to 20 % (Migliavacca et al. 2005). Thereafter, from the insertion till implantation, stents are subjected to conditions as described in Table 3.1.

As the consequence of the mechanical stresses generated by the stent after deployment, remodeling of the arterial wall is occurred (Grewe et al. 2000). The remodeling process can take up to 6–12 months (Grewe et al. 2000; König et al. 2002; Willfort-Ehringer et al. 2004). At the end, the arterial tissue found a new equilibrium where the continued presence of stent is not necessary anymore. Therefore, it may say that the role of stenting is only temporary. Late thrombosis and chronic inflammation could be provoked by the long-term presence of stents (Virmani et al. 2004) and may lead to in-stent restenosis problems (Hoffmann et al. 1996). In paediatric intervention, the disappearing of the stent will easily enable further vessel growth and will avoid the need for further serial stent dilatation to adulthood (Zartner et al. 2005; Schranz et al. 2006). Therefore, biodegradable stents are envisaged to support the arterial wall during the remodeling and to degrade thereafter. The problem of late stent thrombosis is unlikely and the prolonged anti-platelet therapy is not required (Waksman 2006).

Table 3.1 Environmental conditions of implanted coronary stents

Parameters	Values
Blood plasma main composition (Schneck 2000)	Protein: albumin, globulin, fibrinogen
	Ions: chloride, sodium, bicarbonate, etc.
	Lipid : cholesterol, phospholipid, triglyceride
Blood's physical parameters: (Doriot et al. 2000; Muller-Hulsbeck et al. 2001)	
• Density	1.06 g/cm^3
• Viscosity	3–4 mPa.s
• pH	7.4
• Average peak velocity	7–25 cm/s
• Temperature	37 °C
• Shear stress	0.3–1.2 Pa
Dynamic load cycle (Marrey et al. 2006)	10^8 cycles for a 10 year life
Heart beating pressure (Marrey et al. 2006)	Systole: 80 mmHg ($\sim$10 kPa)
	Diastole: 120 mmHg ($\sim$16 kPa)
Typical frequency of heart beat and artery pulse (Marrey et al. 2006)	1.17 Hz
Magnetic field generated during MRI (Roberts and Macgowan 2004)	0.2–3 Tesla

3.2 Proposed Metals for Biodegradable Stent

3.2.1 Iron and its Alloys

Iron widely involves in a large number of Fe containing enzymes and proteins in human body. It involves in the decomposition of lipid, protein and DNA damages due to its reactivity to oxygen molecules which might produce reactive species through Fenton reaction (Mueller et al. 2006). It also plays significant roles in transport, reduction of ribonucleotides and dinitrogen, storage and activation of molecular oxygen, etc. (Fontcave and Pierre 1993).

Pure Fe could be beneficial for human endothelial cell proliferation as the cells were metabolically inhibited only with elution medium in the concentration higher than 50 µg/ml regardless of incubation time (Zhu et al. 2009). An in vitro study reported that excess of Fe ions reduced growth rate of smooth muscle cells which was viewed as positive in term of preventing restenosis in stent application (Mueller et al. 2006). In vivo implantation of pure Fe stents in the descending aorta of New Zealand rabbits has shown preferably results where thromboembolic complications, significant neointimal proliferation, systemic toxicity, pronounced inflammatory response were not observed during the study up to 18 months (Peuster et al. 2001).

Elastic modulus of pure Fe (211.4 GPa) is higher than that of pure Mg (41 GPa) and its alloys (44 GPa) or SS316L (190 GPa) (Song 2007; Sangiorgi et al. 2007). However, Fe is considered as having relatively very slow in vivo degradation rate (Peuster et al. 2006b) and its ferromagnetic nature constitutes a problem as implantable devices. New developed Fe-based alloys have shown a comparable mechanical properties to that of SS316L and has faster degradation rate (0.44 mm/ year) compared to that of pure Fe (Hermawan et al. 2007). These austenitic alloys were a result of alloying Fe with 30–35wt% Mn which turned the alloys into antiferromagnetic. Consequently, the alloys became compatible with magnetic field such as generated from the MRI, a growing non-invasive diagnostic tool in medical imaging.

3.2.2 Magnesium and its Alloys

Magnesium is largely found in bone tissue and is beneficial to bone strength and growth. It is a co-factor for several metabolic enzymes and stabilizes the structure of DNA and RNA (Hartwig 2001). This essential element is the fourth most abundant cation in human body with the daily intake of 300–400 mg in the normal adult (Emsley 1998). Its amount in blood plasma can be tolerated up to a relatively high level of 85–121 mg/l (Saris et al. 2000). Excess Mg level could lead to muscular paralysis, respiratory distress, cardiac arrest and hypotension while its deficiency is reported to cause cell membrane dysfunction, increased incidence of heart disease, cancer and susceptibility to oxidative stress. However, due to the efficient filtration of kidney and excretion in the urine, those are considered be unlikely (Saris et al. 2000; Vormann 2003).

Magnesium and its alloys have been considered to be safe to be fabricated as implantable materials. Their cytocompatibility have been proven by some works including an indirect contact cytotoxicity test involved sterilized pure Mg and Mg–Ca alloys using L-929 cells (Li et al. 2004, 2008) and test on Mg-hydroxy-apatite composite using human bone derived cells and MG-63 plus RAW 264.7 cells (Witte et al. 2007). Other cytotoxicity studies for Mg alloys were also reported (Heublein et al. 2003; Li et al. 2004; Witte et al. 2007; Li et al. 2008).

Orthopaedic implants are the targeted applications of Mg and its alloys due to their supportive physical properties to human bones; i.e. Mg has density near to that of the natural bones (1.8–2 g/cm^3). Pins made of Mg–Ca alloy have been implanted into the rabbit femoral shaft whereas the results showed that the pins were completely degraded within 90 days and followed by the formation of new bone tissue (Li et al. 2004). Other works have also reported that Mg implant supported the activation of bone cells (Witte et al. 2005). The only concern for the use of Mg for orthopaedic implants is their rapid corrosion rate (10–200 mm/year with 99.9 % purity in 3 % NaCl) (Li et al. 2004). Many attempts have been conducted to enhance their corrosion resistance, including by alloying

Table 3.2 Properties of some biodegradable metals compared to SS316L

Metal and its composition (wt%)	Metallurgy	Density (g/cm^3)	Magneticity	YS (MPa)	UTS (MPa)	YM (GPa)	e (%)
WE43 Mg alloy Mg, 3.7–4.3Y, 2.4–4.4Nd, 0.4–1Zr (ASTM 2007)	Hot extruded bar	1.84	NF	150	250	44	4
Pure Fe[a] 99.8Fe	Annealed plate	7.87	FM	150	210	200	40
SS316L (ASTM 2003)	Annealed plate	8.00	NF	190	490	193	40

YS = yield strength, UTS = ultimate tensile strength, YM = Young's modulus, e = maximum elongation, NF = non-ferromagnetic, FM = ferromagnetic
[a] Goodfellow Corporation, Oakdale, PA, USA

(Song 2007), by coating of dicalcium phosphate dehydrate (DCPD) (Wang et al. 2008) and by alkali-heat treatment (Li et al. 2004).

3.3 Mechanical Property of the Proposed Metals

Table 3.2 compares mechanical properties of two biodegradable metals already tested in vivo with SS316L. As the most used medical grade alloy, SS316L is often considered as a standard reference for mechanical properties in developing new metallic biomaterials (Balcon et al. 1997). Pure Fe possesses mechanical properties closer to those of SS316L than Mg alloys which makes Fe preferable for applications that require high strength and ductility such as coronary stents. However, unlike most metallic nonmagnetic biomaterials, Fe is a ferromagnetic substance which may not be preferable in the era of MRI that becomes the default non-invasive imaging modality for coronary investigation.

Compared to most Fe alloys, the ductility of Mg alloys is limited (Mordike and Ebert 2001). However, it can be improved by alloying and employing advanced processing techniques. For example, alloying Mg with Li can change the crystal structure from hexagonal to body centered cubic and produces a large increase in ductility. Alloying with 8.7wt% Li showed 52 % elongation but in exchange, tensile strength dropped to 132 MPa (Sanschagrin et al. 1996). Alloying of Mg may be limited to few metals which are known to be tolerated in the human body, including Ca, Zn, Mn and a very small amount of rare earth elements such as Y and Zr (Song 2007). A slower degradation rate is required to allow the body to regulate OH$^-$ and H$_2$ gas which are usually generated during degradation. Cautions should be taken in designing Mg alloy since the release of alloying elements such as Al, Mn and Zr might induce toxic effect to the body. Aluminum ions have been reported to induce dementia since it might bind to the inorganic phosphate causing the body lack of phosphate source (Lucey and Venugopal 1977). Excess of

Table 3.3 Implantation of metallic biodegradable stents in animal

Material	Implantation site	Finding
Fe (Peuster et al. 2001)	Descending aorta of New Zealand rabbit for 18 months	Lack local or systemic toxicity; low thrombogenicity; mild inflammatory response; accelerated degradation was warranted
AE21 (Heublein et al. 2003)	Coronary artery of pigs for 56 days	Mg alloy stents were promising; prolonged degradation was desired
Fe (Peuster et al. 2006b)	Descending aorta of minipig for 12 months	Neointimal proliferation was comparable to SS316L stent; no local or systemic toxicity; a faster degradation rate was desirable
WE43 (Waksman et al. 2006)	Coronary artery of domestic or minipig for 3 months	Mg alloy stents were safe and associated with less neointima formation; long-term studies (>3 months) were needed to prove positive remodeling
WE43 (Waksman et al. 2007)	Coronary artery of domestic pig with VBT for 28 days	VBT as adjunct to stenting further reduced intimal hyperplasia and improved lumen area when compared to stenting alone
Fe (Waksman et al. 2008)	Coronary arteries of porcine for 28 days	Fe stents were considered safe

Mn also has been reported to cause neurotoxicity that lead to Parkinsinian syndrome (Crossgrove and Zheng 2004). Meanwhile, the presence of Zr is closely associated to the liver, lung, breast and nasopharyngeal cancers (Song 2007).

A hot extruded Mg alloyed with 1wt% Ca showed a good combination of strength and ductility, where tensile strength reached 240 MPa with 11 % elongation (Li et al. 2008). Other processes have reported to improve ductility of Mg alloys including grain refinement (Mukai et al. 2001) and texturing through an equal channel angular processing (ECAP) (Agnew et al. 2004). A recent study on Mg–Zn–Y–Nd alloy made through a cyclic extrusion compression showed an improvement in mechanical properties where it's elongation and yield strength measured at 30.2 % and 185 MPa, respectively (Wu et al. 2012).

3.4 Validation of the Proposed Metals

Initiated by two pioneering works published in early 2000, more in vivo studies have proved the potentiality of biodegradable metals to be used in cardiovascular applications. The first two works are the implantation of Fe stents into the descending aorta of New Zealand white rabbits (Peuster et al. 2001) and the implantation of AE21 Mg alloy stents into the coronary artery of domestic pigs (Heublein et al. 2003) followed by at least four other works on animal studies of metallic biodegradable stents have been published (Table 3.3).

A long-term implantation of Fe stents in the descending aorta of minipigs has shown that there was no difference in the amount of neointimal proliferation between SS316L (control) and Fe stents. Sign of Fe overload or Fe-related organ toxicity was not found as well as any evidence for local toxicity due to corrosion products. Even it was concluded that Fe is a suitable metal for the production of a large-size biodegradable stent, a faster degradation rate was desirable (Peuster et al. 2006b). Assessment of the safety and efficacy of Fe stents was conducted by a short-term implantation of Fe and Co–Cr (control) stents in the coronary arteries of juvenile domestic pigs (Waksman et al. 2008). The results showed that the intimal thickness, intimal area, and percentage of occlusion were better for the Fe stents which lead to a conclusion that Fe stents were relatively safe. The advantage of Fe stents was also mentioned in a study that showed that ions released from the stent could reduce vascular smooth muscle cells (VSMCs) proliferation, an event associated with the problem of in-stent restenosis (Mueller et al. 2006).

The safety and efficacy of Mg alloy stents was assessed by implantation of the stents in porcine coronary arteries where the results lead to a conclusion that Mg alloy stents were safe and were associated with less neointima formation compared to stainless steel stents (Waksman et al. 2006). A follow-up study was conducted involving the use of adjunct vascular brachytherapy (VBT) to overcome the modest degree of late recoil and intimal hyperplasia found in the previous study. It was found that VBT further reduced the intimal hyperplasia and improved the lumen area even though did not improve the late recoil (Waksman et al. 2007). Magnesium alloy stents were even advanced into human assessment which tells us that biodegradable stents are no longer just a concept but reality. Table 3.4 summarizes findings of published reports on implantation trials of Mg alloy stents in human.

Magnesium alloy stents have been reportedly used to treat several clinical cases. In the first case, a preterm baby with a congenital heart disease was treated and the left lung reperfusion was successfully re-established. The stent was proved to be mechanically adequate to secure the reperfusion during 4 months of follow-up while degradation process was clinically well tolerated. Even though the baby died from multiple organ failure after 5 months of implantation, it was an interesting finding that the stent had completely disappeared after 3 months (Zartner et al. 2005). The stent struts were substituted by a jelly-like calcium phosphate and fibrotic structure which allowed a slight increase of the intraluminal diameter over the original stent diameter (Zartner et al. 2007).

In the second case, another newborn with severely impaired heart function due to a long segment recoarctation following a complex surgical repair was also treated with Mg alloy stent where it was able to sustain perfusion without measurable recoil. However, implantation of a second stent was required due to a rapid degradation process that caused the operated vessel backslided into its previous course. Despite the use of two stents, pathological Mg levels in serum were not detected (Schranz et al. 2006).

Table 3.4 Implantation trials of Mg alloy stents in human

Implantation trial	Finding
Pre-clinical testing of stents for CLI in adult patients (Peeters et al. 2005)	3 months primary clinical patency and limb salvage rates suggest a potentially of the stents for CLI treatment
Implantation of stents to treat critical recoarctation of the aorta in a newborn (Schranz et al. 2006)	The stent can be used for the treatment of aortic coarctation in a newborn
Implantation of stents to open an occlusion in the left pulmonary artery of a preterm baby (Zartner et al. 2005; Zartner et al. 2007)	Completed degradation of the stent led to minimal changes within the arterial wall; the stent implantation has rescued a child from an extremely severe clinical problem
Implantation of stents to treat stenotic aorto-pulmonary collateral in a two months old baby girl (McMahon et al. 2007)	There was an initial significant increase in vessel diameter but 4 months after stent placement significant restenosis occurred
PROGRESS-AMS clinical trial (Erbel et al. 2007)	The stents can be safely degraded after 4 months; the immediate angiographic result was similar to the result of other metal stents
AMS-INSIGHT clinical trial (Bosiers et al. 2009)	The stent technology can be safely applied; long-term patency over standard PTA in the infrapopliteal vessels was unclear

In the third case, a 2-month-old girl with pulmonary atresia and hypoplastic pulmonary arteries was also treated with Mg alloy stent where at the beginning there was a significant increase in vessel diameter, but 4 months later, a significant restenosis occurred (McMahon et al. 2007). These cases showed a very promising potential of metallic biodegradable stent for the intervention in children previously deemed unsuitable for permanent stent placement. The latest two cases indicated that further refinement in the Mg alloy stent technology is needed.

More structured human studies of the use of Mg alloy stents were reported. First, a pre-clinical study that use the stent for critical limb ischemia (CLI) treatment in 19 adults reported a high primary clinical patency (89 %) during a preliminary 3-month follow-up. The limb salvage rate was 100 % since no major or minor amputation was necessary in any of the patients thus it was suggested the stents is promising for the treatment of CLI patients (Peeters et al. 2005).

Second report came from a multi-centre, non-randomised prospective study, the PROGRESS-AMS (Clinical Performance and angiographic Results of Coronary Stenting with Absorbable Metal Stents) where 71 stents were successfully implanted in 63 patients. The results showed that the ischaemia-driven target lesion revascularization (TLR) rate was 23.8 % after 4 months and the overall TLR rate was 45 % after one year. It was revealed that Mg alloy stents can achieve an immediate angiographic response similar to that of other metallic stents and be safely degraded after 4 months (Erbel et al. 2007). However, the study suggested that it is necessary to modify the stent characteristics with prolonged degradation time.

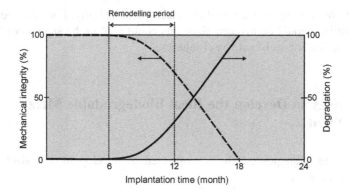

Fig. 3.2 Illustration of an ideal compromise between degradation and mechanical integrity of a biodegradable stent. Adapted with permission from Elsevier (Hermawan et al. 2010)

The latest report came from Absorbable Metal Stent Implantation for Treatment of Below-the-Knee CLI (AMS-INSIGHT) clinical study involving 117 patients with 149 CLI lesions and Mg alloy stenting. The study revealed a comparable complication rate in patients treated with percutaneous transluminal angioplasty (PTA) and PTA + stenting on 30 days follow up, but the 6-month angiographic patency rate in PTA + stenting patients was significantly lower than the rate for those treated with PTA alone (Bosiers et al. 2009). Finally, the study concluded that AMS efficacy in long-term patency over standard PTA in the infrapopliteal vessels was not evident.

3.5 Idealization of Biodegradable Metals for Stent

From the first introduction of the idea of biodegradable stent in 1988 (Stack et al. 1988) until the recent clinical study (Bosiers et al. 2009), we can highlight at least two main characteristics for biodegradable stents to possess:

1. Mechanical properties of the metals pass the minimum value of SS316L to ensure the developed stents to display clinical excellent performances as it has been shown by SS316L stents;
2. Complete degradation occurs after the vessel remodeling process takes place.

An ideal compromise between degradation and mechanical integrity during in vivo implantation as illustrated in Fig. 3.2 should be achieved. It begins at a very slow degradation rate to keep the optimal mechanical integrity during arterial vessel remodeling. Thereafter, the degradation progresses while the mechanical integrity decreases. The degradation ideally occurs at a sufficient rate that will not cause an intolerable accumulation of degradation product around the implantation site. A uniform corrosion mechanism is expected where it begins from the surface to the bulk in order to maintain uniform mechanical integrity. Localized corrosion such as pitting should be avoided since this could lead to the stent's cracking or fragmenting leading to blood vessel injuries.

3.6 Strategy to Develop the Ideal Biodegradable Metals for Stent

At least three strategies can be implemented to develop biodegradable stents having ideal features.

3.6.1 New Alloys Development

Developing new classes of metallic alloys with a broad range of new alloy compositions can be proposed. Even though, the design may be limited by the toxicological consideration of the chosen elements. In today's technology, only Fe and Mg are considered for base metal due to their high limit of toxicity human body (Emsley 1998) and few alloying to chose including Ca, Zn, Mn and a very small amount of REs (Song 2007).

Accordingly, new alloys have been proposed recently, including Mg–Ca alloys (Kannan and Raman 2008; Li et al. 2008) and Mg–Zn/Mn alloys (Song 2007), Fe–Mn–Pd (Schinhammer et al. 2010), Fe–Mn–(Co, C, Al, etc.) plus (Liu and Zheng 2011). In general, those new developed alloys showed improved features in both mechanical properties and degradation behavior, but were not yet tested in vivo.

It has to be emphasized that biodegradable metals might also be coated with degradable polymers or ceramics. By coating, we may target the starting time of the degradation process of the metal. Polymeric coatings can eventually be charged with drugs providing specific targeting effects.

3.6.2 New Processing Technique

Non-conventional processing techniques could improve properties rather than making alloys through traditional melting process. By casting compositional segregation and non-uniform grain structure leading to inferior mechanical properties and degradation behavior are very common.

Two non-conventional processing techniques have been proposed for developing metals for biodegradable stents: powder metallurgy (PM) (Datta et al. 2011; Wegener et al. 2011) and electrodeposition (Moravej et al. 2010a). These methods, mainly electrodeposition, offer an advantage in producing metals with high purity which eliminate the problem of impurities as in the case of cast Mg alloys that lead to a faster and localized degradation.

Heat treatment (Moszner et al. 2011), thermo-mechanical processes, i.e. extrusion (Wang et al. 2011a), and surface modifications constitute conventional but more applicable processes to tailor mechanical properties and degradation behavior of biodegradable metals. Additionally, amorphization of Mg-based (Zberg et al. 2009; Wang et al. 2012), amorphization of Fe-based (Wang et al. 2009) or nanocrystalization of Fe-based alloys (Nie et al. 2010) could be also explored as a potential way to revolutionarily alter the conventional properties of metals.

3.6.3 Iterative Validation Method

Third strategy is by developing validation method which can verify alloy's degradation performance, or even the implant, and give feedback for improvement during design and development cycles. Purnama et al. have proposed a gene-based assessment method to predict cell behavior in the presence of biodegradable metal and its degradation products that are closely related to DNA damage (Purnama et al. 2010). Their method could be very useful for selecting and determining alloying elements and their compositional range.

Pierson et al. have developed a simplified in vivo approach for evaluating bioabsorbable behavior of candidate stent materials (Pierson et al. 2012). This approach can validate in vivo performance of the developed alloy at lower cost and shorter time compared to normal in vivo tests.

Wu et al. have proposed finite element modeling for evaluating degradation of a bioabsorbable stent (Wu et al. 2011). This modeling could effectively match the material properties of an alloy with the structural design of a targeted implant.

References

Agnew SR, Horton JA, Lillo TM, Brown DW (2004) Enhanced ductility in strongly textured magnesium produced by equal channel angular processing. Scr Mater 50:377–381

ASTM (2003) ASTM F 138: standard specification for wrought 18chromium-14nickel-2.5molybdenum stainless steel bar and wire for surgical implants (UNS S31673). ASTM International, West Conshohocken

ASTM (2007) ASTM B 107/B 107 M: specification for magnesium-alloy extruded bars, rods, profiles, tubes, and wire. ASTM International, West Conshohocken

Balcon R, Beyar R, Chierchia S, De Scheerder I, Hugenholtz PG, Kiemeneij F, Meier B, Meyer J, Monassier JP, Wijns W (1997) Recommendations on stent manufacture, implantation and utilization. Eur Heart J 18:1536–1547

Bosiers M, Peeters P, D'Archambeau O, Hendriks J, Pilger E, Duber C, Zeller T, Gussmann A, Lohle PNM, Minar E, Scheinert D, Hausegger K, Schulte K-L, Verbist J, Deloose K, Lammer J

(2009) AMS INSIGHT—absorbable metal stent implantation for treatment of below-the-knee critical limb ischemia: 6-month analysis. Cardiovasc Intervent Radiol 32:424–435

Colombo A, Hall P, Nakamura S, Almagor Y, Maiello L, Martini G, Gaglione A, Goldberg SL, Tobis JM (1995) Intracoronary stenting without anticoagulation accomplished with intravascular ultrasound guidance. Circulation 91:1676–1688

Crossgrove J, Zheng W (2004) Manganese toxicity upon overexposure. NMR Biomed 17:544–553

Datta MK, Chou DT, Hong D, Saha P, Chung SJ, Lee B, Sirinterlikci A, Ramanathan M, Roy A, Kumta PN (2011) Structure and thermal stability of biodegradable Mg–Zn–Ca based amorphous alloys synthesized by mechanical alloying. Mater Sci Eng B 176:1637–1643

Doriot PA, Dorsaz PA, Dorsaz L, De Benedetti E, Chatelain P, Delafontaine P (2000) In vivo measurements of wall shear stress in human coronary arteries. Coron Artery Dis 11:495–502

Elliot JS, Ajay K, Martin TR (2006) New developments in coronary stent technology. J Interv Cardiol 19:493–499

Emsley J (1998) The elements. Clarendon Press, Oxford

Erbel R, Di Mario C, Bartunek J, Bonnier J, de Bruyne B, Eberli FR, Erne P, Haude M, Heublein B, Horrigan M, Ilsley C, Bose D, Koolen J, Luscher TF, Weissman N, Waksman R (2007) Temporary scaffolding of coronary arteries with bioabsorbable magnesium stents: a prospective, non-randomised multicentre trial. Lancet 369:1869–1875

Fischman DL, Leon MB, Baim DS, Schatz RA, Savage MP, Penn I, Detre K, Veltri L, Ricci D, Nobuyoshi M et al (1994) A randomized comparison of coronary-stent placement and balloon angioplasty in the treatment of coronary artery disease. Stent restenosis study investigators. N Engl J Med 331:496–501

Fontcave M, Pierre JL (1993) Iron: metabolism, toxicity and therapy. Biochimie 73:767–773

Grewe PH, Thomas D, Machraoui A, Barmeyer J, Muller KM (2000) Coronary morphologic findings after stent implantation. Am J Cardiol 85:554–558

Hartwig A (2001) Role of magnesium in genomic stability. Mutat Res 475:113–121

Hermawan H, Moravej M, Dube D, Mantovani D (2007) Degradation behaviour of metallic biomaterials for degradable stents. Adv Mater Res 15–17:113–118

Hermawan H, Dube D, Mantovani D (2010) Developments in metallic biodegradable stents. Acta Biomater 6:1693–1697

Heublein B, Rohde R, Kaese V, Niemeyer M, Hartung W, Haverich A (2003) Biocorrosion of magnesium alloys: a new principle in cardiovascular implant technology? Heart 89:651–656

Hoffmann R, Mintz GS, Dussaillant GR, Popma JJ, Pichard AD, Satler LF, Kent KM, Griffin J, Leon MB (1996) Patterns and mechanisms of in-stent restenosis. A serial intravascular ultrasound study. Circulation 94:1247–1254

Kannan MB, Raman RKS (2008) In vitro degradation and mechanical integrity of calcium-containing magnesium alloys in modified-simulated body fluid. Biomaterials 29:2306–2314

King SB, Hirshfeld JW, Williams DO, Feldman TE, Kern MJ, O'Neill WW, Williams DO, Jacobs AK, Buller CE, Hunt SA, Lytle BW, Tarkington LG, Yancy CW (2008) 2007 focused update of the ACC/AHA/SCAI 2005 guideline update for percutaneous coronary intervention. Circulation 117:261–295

König A, Schiele TM, Rieber J, Theisen K, Mudra H, Klauss V (2002) Influence of stent design and deployment technique on neointima formation and vascular remodeling. Z Kardiol 91:98–102

Li L, Gao J, Wang Y (2004) Evaluation of cyto-toxicity and corrosion behavior of alkali-heat-treated magnesium in simulated body fluid. Surf Coat Technol 185:92–98

Li Z, Gu X, Lou S, Zheng Y (2008) The development of binary Mg–Ca alloys for use as biodegradable materials within bones. Biomaterials 29:1329–1344

Liu B, Zheng YF (2011) Effects of alloying elements (Mn, Co., Al, W, Sn, B, C and S) on biodegradability and in vitro biocompatibility of pure iron. Acta Biomater 7:1407–1420

Lucey TD, Venugopal B (1977) Metal toxicity in mammals. Plenum Press, New York

Marrey RV, Burgermeister R, Grishaber RB, Ritchie RO (2006) Fatigue and life prediction for cobalt-chromium stents: a fracture mechanics analysis. Biomaterials 27:1988–2000

McMahon CJ, Oslizlok P, Walsh KP (2007) Early restenosis following biodegradable stent implantation in an aortopulmonary collateral of a patient with pulmonary atresia and hypoplastic pulmonary arteries. Catheter Cardiovasc Interv 69:735–738

Migliavacca F, Petrini L, Montanari V, Quagliana I, Auricchio F, Dubini G (2005) A predictive study of the mechanical behaviour of coronary stents by computer modelling. Med Eng Phys 27:13–18

Moravej M, Prima F, Fiset M, Mantovani D (2010) Electroformed iron as new biomaterial for degradable stents: development process and structure-properties relationship. Acta Biomater 6:1726–1735

Mordike BL, Ebert T (2001) Magnesium properties, applications and potential. Mater Sci Eng A 302:37–45

Moszner F, Sologubenko AS, Schinhammer M, Lerchbacher C, Hänzi AC, Leitner H, Uggowitzer PJ, Löffler JF (2011) Precipitation hardening of biodegradable Fe–Mn–Pd alloys. Acta Mater 59:981–991

Mueller PP, May T, Perz A, Hauser H, Peuster M (2006) Control of smooth muscle cell proliferation by ferrous iron. Biomaterials 27(10):2193–2200

Mukai T, Yamanoi M, Watanabe H, Higashi K (2001) Ductility enhancement in AZ31 magnesium alloy by controlling its grain structure. Scr Mater 45:89–94

Muller-Hulsbeck S, Grimm J, Jahnke T, Haselbarth G, Heller M (2001) Flow patterns from metallic vascular endoprostheses: in vitro results. Eur Radiol 11:893–901

Nie FL, Zheng YF, Wei SC, Hu C, Yang G (2010) In vitro corrosion, cytotoxicity and hemocompatibility of bulk nanocrystalline pure iron. Biomed Mater 5:065015

Peeters P, Bosiers M, Verbist J, Deloose K, Heublein B (2005) Preliminary results after application of absorbable metal stents in patients with critical limb ischemia. J Endovasc Ther 12:1–5

Peuster M, Wohlsein P, Brugmann M, Ehlerding M, Seidler K, Fink C, Brauer H, Fischer A, Hausdorf G (2001) A novel approach to temporary stenting: degradable cardiovascular stents produced from corrodible metal-results 6–18 months after implantation into New Zealand white rabbits. Heart 86:563–569

Peuster M, Beerbaum P, Bach FW, Hauser H (2006a) Are resorbable implants about to become a reality? Cardiol Young 16:107–116

Peuster M, Hesse C, Schloo T, Fink C, Beerbaum P, Schnakenburg CV (2006b) Long term biocompatibility of a corrodible peripheral iron stent in the porcine descending aorta. Biomaterials 27:4955–4962

Pierson D, Edick J, Tauscher A, Pokorney E, Bowen P, Gelbaugh J, Stinson J, Getty H, Lee CH, Drelich J, Goldman J (2012) A simplified in vivo approach for evaluating the bioabsorbable behavior of candidate stent materials. J Biomed Mater Res B 100:58–67

Purnama A, Hermawan H, Couet J, Mantovani D (2010) Assessing the biocompatibility of degradable metallic materials: state of the art and focus on the genetic regulation potential. Acta Biomater 6:1800–1807

Roberts TPL, Macgowan CK (2004) Magnetic resonance imaging. In: Moore J, Zouridakis G (eds) Biomedical technology and devices handbook. CRC Press, Boca Raton

Sangiorgi G, Melzi G, Agostoni P, Cola C, Clementi F, Romitelli P, Virmani R, Colombo A (2007) Engineering aspects of stents design and their translation into clinical practice. Ann Ist Super Sanità 43:89–100

Sanschagrin A, Tremblay R, Angers R (1996) Mechanical properties and microstructure of new magnesium-lithium base alloys. Mater Sci Eng 220:69–77

Saris NE, Mervaala E, Karppanen H, Khawaja JA, Lewenstam A (2000) Magnesium. An update on physiological, clinical and analytical aspects. Clin Chim Acta 294:1–26

Schinhammer M, Hänzi AC, Löffler JF, Uggowitzer PJ (2010) Design strategy for biodegradable Fe-based alloys for medical applications. Acta Biomater 6:1705–1713

Schneck DJ (2000) An outline of cardiovascular structure and function. In: Bronzino JD (ed) The biomedical engineering handbook, vol 1, 2nd edn. CRC Press, Boca Raton

Schranz D, Zartner P, Michel-Behnke I, Akinturk H (2006) Bioabsorbable metal stents for percutaneous treatment of critical recoarctation of the aorta in a newborn. Catheter Cardiovasc Interv 67:671–673

Serruys PW, de Jaegere P, Kiemeneij F, Macaya C, Rutsch W, Heyndrickx G, Emanuelsson H, Marco J, Legrand V, Materne P, Belardi J, Sigwart U, Colombo A, Goy JJ, van den Heuvel P, Delcan J, Morel M-A (1994) A comparison of balloon-expandable-stent implantation with balloon angioplasty in patients with coronary artery disease. Benestent study group. N Engl J Med 331:489–495

Serruys PW, Kutryk MJ, Ong AT (2006) Coronary-artery stents. N Engl J Med 354:483–495

Sigwart U, Puel J, Mirkovitch V, Joffre F, Kappenberger L (1987) Intravascular stents to prevent occlusion and restenosis after transluminal angioplasty. N Engl J Med 316:701–706

Song G (2007) Control of biodegradation of biocompatible magnesium alloys. Corr Sci 49:1696–1701

Stack RS, Califf RM, Phillips HR, Pryor DB, Quigley PJ, Bauman RP, Tcheng JE, Greenfield JC Jr (1988) Interventional cardiac catheterization at Duke medical center. Am J Cardiol 62:3F–24F

Virmani R, Farb A, Guagliumi G, Kolodgie FD (2004) Drug-eluting stents: caution and concerns for long-term outcome. Coron Artery Dis 15:313–318

Vormann J (2003) Magnesium: nutrition and metabolism. Mol Aspects Med 24:27–37

Waksman R (2006) Update on bioabsorbable stents: from bench to clinical. J Interv Cardiol 19:414–421

Waksman R (2007) Promise and challenges of bioabsorbable stents. Catheter Cardiovasc Interv 70:407–414

Waksman R, Pakala R, Kuchulakanti PK, Baffour R, Hellinga D, Seabron R, Tio FO, Wittchow E, Hartwig S, Harder C, Rohde R, Heublein B, Andreae A, Waldmann K-H, Haverich A (2006) Safety and efficacy of bioabsorbable magnesium alloy stents in porcine coronary arteries. Catheter Cardiovasc Interv 68:606–617

Waksman R, Pakala R, Okabe T, Hellinga D, Chan R, Tio MO, Wittchow E, Hartwig S, Waldmann KH, Harder C (2007) Efficacy and safety of absorbable metallic stents with adjunct intracoronary beta radiation in porcine coronary arteries. J Interv Cardiol 20:367–372

Waksman R, Pakala R, Baffour R, Seabron R, Hellinga D, Tio FO (2008) Short-term effects of biocorrodible iron stents in porcine coronary arteries. J Interv Cardiol 21:15–20

Wang Y, Wei M, Gao J (2008) Improve corrosion resistance of magnesium in simulated body fluid by dicalcium phosphate dihydrate coating. Mater Sci Eng C 29:1311–1316

Wang YB, Li HF, Cheng Y, Wei SC, Zheng YF (2009) Corrosion performances of a Nickel-free Fe-based bulk metallic glass in simulated body fluids. Electrochem Comm 11:2187–2190

Wang B, Guan S, Wang J, Wang L, Zhu S (2011) Effects of Nd on microstructures and properties of extruded Mg–2Zn–0.46Y–xNd alloys for stent application. Mater Sci Eng B 176:1673–1678

Wang Y, Tan MJ, Jarfors AWE (2012) Corrosion behavior and surface analysis of melt-spun Mg-based metallic glass in physiological saline solution. Mater Sci Forum 706–709:606–611

Wegener B, Sievers B, Utzschneider S, Müller P, Jansson V, Rößler S, Nies B, Stephani G, Kieback B, Quadbeck P (2011) Microstructure, cytotoxicity and corrosion of powder-metallurgical iron alloys for biodegradable bone replacement materials. Mater Sci Eng B 176:1789–1796

Willfort-Ehringer A, Ahmadi R, Gruber D, Gschwandtner ME, Haumer A, Haumer M, Ehringer H (2004) Arterial remodeling and hemodynamics in carotid stents: a prospective duplex ultrasound study over 2 years. J Vasc Surg 39:728–734

Witte F, Kaese V, Haferkamp H, Switzer E, Linderberg AM, Wirth CJ, Windhagen H (2005) In vivo corrosion of four magnesium alloys and the associated bone response. Biomaterials 26:3557–3563

Witte F, Feyerabend F, Maier P, Fischer J, Störmer M, Blawert C, Dietzel W, Hort N (2007) Biodegradable magnesium-hydroxyapatite metal matrix composites. Biomaterials 28:2163–2174

Wu W, Gastaldi D, Yang K, Tan L, Petrini L, Migliavacca F (2011) Finite element analyses for design evaluation of biodegradable magnesium alloy stents in arterial vessels. Mater Sci Eng B 176:1733–1740

Wu Q, Zhu S, Wang L, Liu Q, Yue G, Wang J, Guan S (2012) The microstructure and properties of cyclic extrusion compression treated Mg–Zn–Y–Nd alloy for vascular stent application. J Mech Behav Biomed Mater 8:1–7

Zartner P, Cesnjevar R, Singer H, Weyand M (2005) First successful implantation of a biodegradable metal stent into the left pulmonary artery of a preterm baby. Catheter Cardiovasc Interv 66:590–594

Zartner P, Buettner M, Singer H, Sigler M (2007) First biodegradable metal stent in a child with congenital heart disease: evaluation of macro and histopathology. Catheter Cardiovasc Interv 69:443–446

Zberg B, Uggowitzer PJ, Loffler JF (2009) MgZnCa glasses without clinically observable hydrogen evolution for biodegradable implants. Nat Mater 8:887–891

Zhu S, Huang N, Xu L, Zhang Y, Liu H, Sun H, Leng Y (2009) Biocompatibility of pure iron: in vitro assessment of degradation kinetics and cytotoxicity on endothelial cells. Mater Sci Eng C 29:1589–1592

Chapter 4
Metallic Biodegradable Coronary Stent: Materials Development

Abstract By taking 316L stainless steel as reference for mechanical and physical properties, a series of iron-manganese alloys was developed. Four alloys with manganese content ranging from 20 to 35wt% were prepared. Their microstructure, mechanical and physical properties were carefully investigated. Results show that the developed alloys possess mechanical and physical properties suitable for the development of biodegradable coronary stents.

Keywords Biodegradable stent · Fe-Mn alloy · Mechanical property · Magnetic property · Powder metallurgy

4.1 Materials Design

As derived from the Fig. 3.2, three design criteria have been determined for developing new alloys for biodegradable stent: (1) mechanical properties that approach to those of SS316L; (2) degradation rate that matches with vessel remodeling period (6–12 months) (Schomig et al. 1994) and complete disappearance of the implant material within a reasonable period (12–24 months) (Serruys et al. 2006); and (3) no toxic substances are released during the degradation process.

Iron was viewed as more attractive than Mg alloys considering its superior mechanical properties in regard to those of SS316L (Table 3.2). A proper alloying and thermo-mechanical treatment could further enhance the properties of Fe. A careful selection of alloying elements could also transform the ferromagnetism of Fe into nonmagnetism, thus providing a good compatibility with magnetic field such as generated during MRI procedure.

Based on an extensive materials analysis and toxicological review on potential alloying elements for Fe, the choice was narrowed to Mn which can turn Fe into

H. Hermawan, *Biodegradable Metals*, SpringerBriefs in Materials, DOI: 10.1007/978-3-642-31170-3_4, © The Author(s) 2012

Fig. 4.1 Phase diagram of
binary Fe-Mn system.
Adapted with permission
from the Iron and Steel
Institute of Japan (Lee et al.
1997)

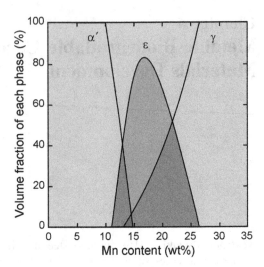

nonmagnetic, known as austenite-forming element (Hansen 1958; Huang 1989).
Figure 4.1 shows Fe-Mn alloy phase diagram. Nickel is also an austenite forming
element but it can form compounds classified as carcinogenic to human (Boffetta
1993; McGregor et al. 2000). Manganese is an essential trace element for the body
function of all mammals (Keen et al. 2000). Its excess was not reported to be toxic
in cardiovascular system due to the extensive plasma protein binding counteract
the effect of Mn toxicity (Jynge et al. 1997; Crossgrove and Zheng 2004).

Austenitic (γ) phase starts to form at about 15wt% Mn content mixed with
martensite (ε) up to about 27wt% Mn and thereafter only γ should be present (Lee
et al. 1997). The ε and γ phases possess antiferromagnetic properties (Ishikawa and
Endoh 1968; Rabinkin 1979) that allow Fe-Mn alloys containing exclusively these
phases to be nonmagnetic. Therefore, alloys containing 20–35wt% Mn were
prepared and evaluated for their potentiality as biodegradable stent materials.

4.2 Materials Production

Four Fe-Mn alloys, namely Fe-20Mn, Fe-25Mn, Fe-30Mn and Fe-35Mn, were
produced from high purity elemental powders (purity 99.98 %) of Fe and Mn.
Powder metallurgy was selected to fabricate the alloys to ensure high-purity and
homogenous composition while also provide porosity for degradation control.
Powder mixtures were compacted and sintered in a flowing Ar-5 %H_2 gas mixture
at 1200 °C for 3 h. Figure 4.2 shows the alloys production process flow chart,
additional details were reported elsewhere (Hermawan et al. 2007, 2008).

Two steps of thermo-mechanical treatment were then applied to the sintered
pellets to obtain high density material with aligned porosity: (1) cold rolled by
50 % thickness reduction and resintered at 1200 °C for 2 h and furnace cooling;

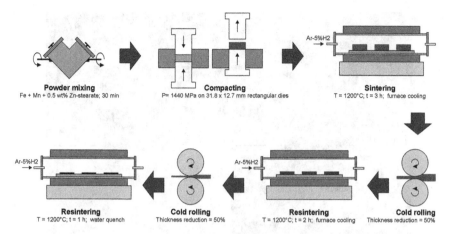

Fig. 4.2 Schematic process flow chart for Fe-Mn alloy production

(2) cold rolled by another 50 % thickness reduction and resintered at 1200 °C for 1 h then water quenched. The aligned porosity was expected to act as a physical barrier controlling the degradation rate.

4.3 Microstructure Analysis

The produced alloys contained negligible amount of C, Si and N, therefore their known influence to martensitic transformations (i.e. $\gamma \rightarrow \varepsilon$ and $\gamma \rightarrow \alpha'$) in Fe-Mn alloys (Bogachev et al. 1969; Zvigintseva et al. 1970; Bliznuk et al. 2002) can be neglected. Moreover, their effect was diminished by the relatively high Mn content where nominally the alloys contained of: 18.4wt% (Fe20Mn), 24.0wt% (Fe-25Mn), 19.3wt% (Fe-30Mn) and 35.3wt% (Fe-35Mn) of Mn, respectively.

The cold rolling and resintering process allowed pores and inclusion to be aligned along rolling direction. Porosity was gradually reduced down to less than 1 % at the end of the process. As in the case of roll compacted Fe-Al foils (Deevi 2000), the densification was suggested due to pores reconfiguration aided by recrystallization (Volynova et al. 1992). Typical microstructure of the produced Fe-Mn alloys is shown in Fig. 4.3.

The microstructure consists essentially of equiaxial grains (about 50 μm in diameter) with fine pores and inclusions. In Fe-20Mn and Fe-25Mn (Figs. 4.3a, b), the matrix consists of triangular structures indicating the presence of γ and ε phases (Lee et al. 1997; Schumann 1975), whereas for Fe-30Mn and Fe-35Mn (Figs. 4.3c, d) only γ phase presents. X-ray diffraction (XRD) spectra confirmed the presence of γ and ε phases in Fe-20Mn and Fe-25Mn, and only γ phase were detected in Fe-30Mn and Fe-35Mn. Their presence was just as expected from Fig. 4.1, where similar finding were also obtained in other works (Lee et al. 1997; Martinez et al. 2005).

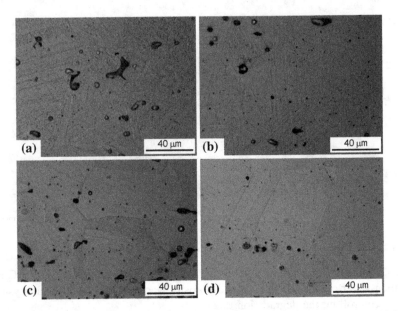

Fig. 4.3 Typical microstructure of the produced: **a** Fe-20Mn, **b** Fe-25Mn, **c** Fe-30Mn, and **d** Fe-35Mn. Adapted with permission from John Wiley and Sons (Hermawan et al. 2010)

Interestingly in Fe-Mn system, a martensitic $\gamma \rightarrow \varepsilon$ transformation occurred under the influence of plastic deformation (Bogachev et al. 1972). In Fe-30Mn and Fe-35Mn, γ phase was transformed into ε phase during cold rolling; meanwhile in Fe-20Mn and Fe-25Mn, ε phase has already appeared before. Other works also reported similar results where the presence of ε phase after deformation was stronger in alloys containing relatively less Mn (Bogachev et al. 1972; Gauzzi et al. 1983).

Plastic deformation increases the driving force for martensitic transformation (Cotes et al. 2004) and acts as nucleation site generator (Olson and Cohen 1975) where new stacking faults form and at the same time the ε phase grows by shear-assisted slip mechanism (Trichter et al. 1978). Differently, in cast and homogenized alloys containing more than 30wt% Mn, the formation of ε phase due to plastic deformation was hardly accomplished (Trichter et al. 1978). Porosity was suspected to act as free surface for stress relaxation that could lower the driving force of the transformation where similar effect was observed in Fe-Mn alloys (Gartstein and Rabinkin 1979) and Fe-Ni alloys (Nishiyama and Shimizu 1961).

4.4 Mechanical Property

The Fe-25Mn has the highest ultimate strength than others, while the highest yield strength was obtained by Fe-20Mn specimens. The longest elongation was obtained with Fe-35Mn specimens. Compared to the minimum requirement of

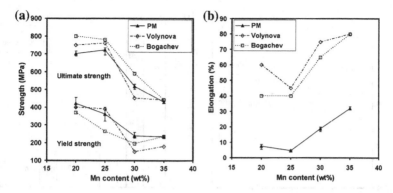

Fig. 4.4 Comparison of: **a** tensile and yield strength, and **b** elongation of Fe-Mn developed by PM to the cast counterparts developed in (Bogachev et al. 1972; Volynova 1984). Adapted with permission from John Wiley and Sons (Hermawan et al. 2010)

ASTM F138 for SS316L, mechanical properties of the Fe-Mn alloys are superior except for elongation. The phase composition strongly influenced the mechanical properties of Fe-Mn alloys. In Fe-20Mn and Fe-25Mn specimens, two $\gamma + \varepsilon$ phases coexisted, while only γ phase wass found in Fe-30Mn and Fe-35Mn specimens. The hard and dense ε phase (Trichter et al. 1978) should be responsible for strengthening the alloys which imply a decrease in strength and an increase in ductility as Mn content increase.

Figure 4.4 compares mechanical property of the produced Fe-Mn alloys to their cast counterparts. It shows that the produced alloys have comparable strength to those of cast studied in previous works (Bogachev et al. 1972; Volynova 1984). However, as expected the maximum elongation is lower than those of the cast counterparts which are ascribed at least in part to the presence of more inclusion and pores in the PM alloys.

Ductility of Fe-20Mn was unexpectedly slight higher than Fe-25Mn, but could be explained by considering the stress relaxation mechanism produced by formation of new phase and deformation twinning (Strudel 1996). Even ε phase was formed in both alloys during tensile test; α' phase was also formed in Fe-20Mn which allowed stress relaxation that in turn extended its elongation. Even though they have the same γ phase, elongation was found to be significantly higher in Fe-35Mn than in Fe-30Mn. The $\gamma \rightarrow \varepsilon$ transformation once again explains well as Fe30Mn has higher sensitivity to the transformation, more ε phase was formed than in Fe-35Mn. The $\gamma-\varepsilon$ interfaces acted as effective barrier to shear propagation (Lee et al. 1997) that in turn provided an increase in strength and decrease in ductility.

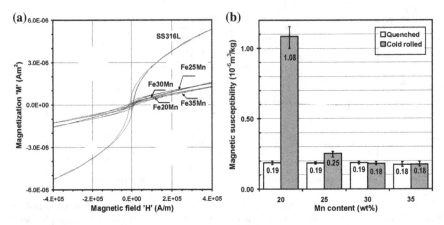

Fig. 4.5 **a** Magnetization curves of Fe-Mn and SS316L, **b** magnetic susceptibility of Fe-Mn after quenched and after cold rolled with 20 % thickness reduction. Adapted with permission from John Wiley and Sons (Hermawan et al. 2010)

4.5 Magnetic Property

Figure 4.5a presents magnetization (hysteresis) curves of the produced Fe-Mn alloys where all curves show positive paramagnetism M/H slopes. It is shown also that as Mn content increases the slopes and the area of hysterisis loops decrease. As derived from the curves, the Fe-Mn alloys possessed lower initial susceptibility compared to SS316L. This could be attributed to the fact that both of γ and ε phases in Fe-Mn alloys are antiferromagnetic (Ishikawa and Endoh 1968; Rabinkin 1979), meanwhile the γ phase in SS316L is paramagnetic.

Figure 4.5b plots magnetic susceptibility of Fe-Mn alloys under quenched and deformed condition against Mn content. It shows that except for Fe-20Mn, magnetic susceptibility of the alloys remained unchanged. Presence of ferromagnetic α' phase formed during plastic deformation was suspected as the reason for the increase of magnetic susceptibility in Fe-20Mn which is supported by several studies on austenitic stainless steel that showed an increase in magnetic susceptibility due $\gamma \rightarrow \alpha'$ transformation when plastically deformed at room temperature (Meszaros and Prohaszka 2005; Mumtaz et al. 2004). Interestingly, the constant magnetic susceptibility will ensures a consistent MRI compatibility of an implant that is deformed during its implantation like a coronary stent.

4.6 Conclusion and Benchmarking

The work was considered as the first that design and develop biomaterials based on a set of criteria translated from clinical needs. It was not just trivially taking excellent materials from other applications and validating their suitability for

Table 4.1 Mechanical properties of Fe-based biodegradable metals

Metal	Metallurgy	Yield strength (MPa)	Tensile strength (MPa)	Elongation (%)
Fe-35Mn (Hermawan et al. 2008)	Thermomechanically treated PM alloy	230	430	30
Fe-10Mn-1Pd (Schinhammer et al. 2010)	Heat treated cast alloy	850–950	1450–1550	2–8
Fe-X (Liu and Zheng 2011)	Cast	100–220	190–360	12–23
Fe-30Mn-6Si (Liu et al. 2011)	Solution treated cast	180	450	16
Fe (Moravej et al. 2010)	Annealed electroformed	270	290	18
Fe (Nie et al. 2010)	ECAP	N/A	250–450	N/A

biomaterials applications. The work has successfully developed four Fe-Mn alloys via PM process followed by a series of resintering and cold rolling treatment. The higher Mn content alloys consisted of essentially austenitic phase and additional epsilon phase was found in lower Mn content alloys. The alloys possessed comparable tensile strength to SS316L but with lower ductility due to retained porosity and formed inclusion. The alloys showed interesting magnetic property where their magnetic susceptibility was lower than SS316L and it was not increased by plastic deformation. It can be concluded that the mechanical and physical property of the developed Fe-Mn alloys are suitable for the development of biodegradable coronary stents.

Recent works on Fe-based alloys have mostly contributed to the improvement of mechanical performance of the previously developed binary Fe-Mn alloys (Hermawan et al. 2010). Table 4.1 summarizes mechanical properties of Fe-based biodegradable metals providing more alternative alloys for biodegradable medical applications.

Following the binary Fe-Mn alloy work (Hermawan et al. 2008), Schinhammer et al. have proposed a design strategy for the development of new biodegradable Fe-based alloys based on toxicological, microstructural and electrochemical considerations (Schinhammer et al. 2010). They modified the electrochemical of the Fe matrix by deployed a controlled formation of noble intermetallic phases by adding Mn and Pd where a formation of (Fe, Mn)Pd intermetallics act as cathodic sites. As the result, the newly developed Fe-Mn-Pd alloys revealed a one order of magnitude lower degradation resistance compared to pure Fe, and a tremendous increase in the mechanical performance following heat treatment procedures, where strength values >1400 MPa at ductility levels >10 % was achieved. Xu et al. have added carbon to binary Fe-Mn alloy to fabricate Fe-30Mn-1C alloy by vacuum induction melting (Xu et al. 2011). They demonstrated that due to the addition of C, the Fe-30Mn-1C alloy had better mechanical properties than those of Fe-30Mn alloy and SS316L with lower magnetic susceptibility and higher degradation rate compared with Fe-30Mn alloy.

Recently, Liu et al. have explored a set of Fe-X binary alloy models where a wide range of alloying elements: Mn, Co, Al, W, B, C and S, and one detrimental impurity element: Sn, was studied (Liu and Zheng 2011). It was shown that the addition of all alloying elements except for Sn improved the mechanical properties of Fe after rolling, and except for the Fe-Mn, which showed a significant decrease in corrosion rate, the other Fe-X binary alloy corrosion rates were close to that of pure Fe. The work then recommended Co, W, C and S as alloying elements for biodegradable Fe-based biomaterials. Another work by the same group has investigated Fe-30Mn-6Si shape memory alloy (Liu et al. 2011). The alloy consisted of ε-martensite and γ-austenite at room temperature, resulting higher mechanical property and degradation rate than those of pure Fe. Having a shape memory function, they conclude Fe-30Mn-6Si alloy to be a promising biodegradable metallic material.

Moravej et al. have worked on pure Fe but with new interesting technique where electroforming was developed for fabricating Fe foils targeted for application as biodegradable cardiovascular stent material (Moravej et al. 2010). The foils possessed fine grain (4 µm) resulting in a high yield (360 MPa) and ultimate tensile strength (423 MPa). Their ductility was increased from 8 to 18 % by annealing at 550 °C. Compared to conventional cast pure Fe, the electroformed Fe showed higher degradation rate. With their fine-grain microstructure, suitable mechanical properties and moderate corrosion rate, the electroformed Fe was considered as a suitable biodegradable stent material. Another different technique was employed by Nie et al. where pure Fe was developed in the form of nanocrystalline rods by the ECAP process (Nie et al. 2010). However, except for tensile strength, degradation rate was not improved.

References

Bliznuk VV, Glavatska NI, Soderberg O, Lindroos VK (2002) Effect of nitrogen on damping, mechanical and corrosive properties of Fe-Mn alloys. Mater Sci Eng A 338:213–218

Boffetta P (1993) Carcinogenicity of trace elements with reference to evaluations made by the International Agency for Research on cancer. Scand J Work Environ Health 19(Suppl 1):67–70

Bogachev IN, Yegolayev VF, Zvigintseva GY, Zhuravel LV (1969) Effect of alloying on austenite imperfection and tendency of an Fe-Mn alloy to γ–ε transformation. Phys Met Metallogr 28:125–130

Bogachev IN, Yegolayev VF, Frolova TL (1972) Features of the strengthening of austenitic iron-manganese alloys. Phys Met Metallogr 33:127–132

Cotes SM, Guillermet AF, Sade M (2004) FCC–HCP martensitic transformation in the Fe-Mn system: Part II. Driving force and thermodynamic of the nucleation process. Metall Mater Trans A 35:83–91

Crossgrove J, Zheng W (2004) Manganese toxicity upon overexposure. NMR Biomed 17:544–553

Deevi SC (2000) Powder processing of FeAl sheets by roll compaction. Intermetallics 8:679–685

Gartstein E, Rabinkin A (1979) On the FCC–HCP phase transformation in high manganese-iron alloys. Acta Metall 27:1053–1064

Gauzzi F, Verdini B, Principi G, Badan B (1983) The martensitic transformation in cold-worked Fe-Mn alloys studied by Mossbauer spectroscopy. J Mater Sci 18:3661–3670

Hansen M (1958) Constitution of binary alloys. McGraw-Hill, Toronto

Hermawan H, Dube D, Mantovani D (2007) Development of degradable Fe-35Mn alloy for biomedical application. Adv Mater Res 15–17:107–112

Hermawan H, Alamdari H, Mantovani D, Dubé D (2008) Iron-manganese: new class of degradable metallic biomaterials prepared by powder metallurgy. Powder Metall 51:38–45

Hermawan H, Dube D, Mantovani D (2010) Degradable metallic biomaterials: design and development of Fe-Mn alloys for stents. J Biomed Mater Res A 93:11

Huang W (1989) An assessment of the Fe-Mn system. Calphad 13:243–252

Ishikawa Y, Endoh Y (1968) Antiferromagnetism of γ-FeMn alloys. J Appl Phys 39:1318–1319

Jynge P, Brurok H, Asplund A, Towart R, Refsum H, Karlsson JO (1997) Cardiovascular safety of MnDPDP and $MnCl_2$. Acta Radiol 38:740–749

Keen CL, Ensunsa JL, Clegg MS (2000) Manganese metabolism in animals and humans including the toxicity of manganese. In: Siegel A, Siegel H (eds) Manganese and its role in biological processes. Marcel Dekker, New York, pp 89–121

Lee Y-K, Jun J-H, Choi C-S (1997) Damping capacity in Fe-Mn binary alloys. ISIJ Int 37:1023–1030

Liu B, Zheng YF (2011) Effects of alloying elements (Mn, Co., Al, W, Sn, B, C and S) on biodegradability and in vitro biocompatibility of pure iron. Acta Biomater 7:1407–1420

Liu B, Zheng YF, Ruan L (2011) In vitro investigation of Fe30Mn6Si shape memory alloy as potential biodegradable metallic material. Mater Lett 65:540–543

Martinez J, Cotes SM, Cabrera AF, Desimoni J, Fernandez Guillermet A (2005) On the relative fraction of epsilon-martensite in gamma-austenite Fe-Mn alloys. Mater Sci Eng A 408:26–32

McGregor DB, Baan RA, Partensky C, Rice JM, Wilbourn JD (2000) Evaluation of the carcinogenic risks to humans associated with surgical implants and other foreign bodies—a report of an IARC Monographs Programme Meeting. Eur J Cancer 36:307–313

Meszaros I, Prohaszka J (2005) Magnetic investigation of the effect of α'-martensite on the properties of austenitic stainless steel. J Mater Proc Technol 161:162–168

Moravej M, Prima F, Fiset M, Mantovani D (2010) Electroformed iron as new biomaterial for degradable stents: development process and structure-properties relationship. Acta Biomater 6:1726–1735

Mumtaz K, Takahashi S, Echigoya J, Kamada Y, Zhang LF, Kikuchi H, Ara K, Sato M (2004) Magnetic measurements of martensitic transformation in austenitic stainless steel after room temperature rolling. J Mater Sci 39:85–97

Nie FL, Zheng YF, Wei SC, Hu C, Yang G (2010) In vitro corrosion, cytotoxicity and hemocompatibility of bulk nanocrystalline pure iron. Biomed Mater 5:065015

Nishiyama Z, Shimizu K (1961) Study of sub-structures of the martensite in Fe-Ni alloy by means of transmission electron microscope. Acta Metall 9:980–981

Olson GB, Cohen M (1975) Kinetics of strain-induced martensitic nucleation. Metall Trans A 6:791–795

Rabinkin A (1979) On magnetic contributions to γ-ε phase transformations in Fe-Mn alloys. Calphad 3:77–84

Schinhammer M, Hänzi AC, Löffler JF, Uggowitzer PJ (2010) Design strategy for biodegradable Fe-based alloys for medical applications. Acta Biomater 6:1705–1713

Schomig A, Kastrati A, Mudra H, Blasini R, Schuhlen H, Klauss V, Richardt G, Neumann FJ (1994) Four-year experience with Palmaz-Schatz stenting in coronary angioplasty complicated by dissection with threatened or present vessel closure. Circulation 90:2716–2724

Schumann H (1975) The influence of mechanical stresses on the microstructures of alloys undergoing the martensitic transformation. Pract Metallogr 12:511–525

Serruys PW, Kutryk MJ, Ong AT (2006) Coronary-artery stents. N Engl J Med 354:483–495

Strudel J-L (1996) Mechanical properties of multiphase alloys. In: Cahn RW (ed) Physical metallurgy, vol III. North-Holland, Amsterdam

Trichter F, Rabinkin A, Ron M, Sharfstein A (1978) A study of gamma-epsilon phase transformation in Fe-Mn alloys induced by high pressure and plastic deformation. Scr Metall 12:431–434

Volynova TF (1984) Nickel-free iron-manganese alloys. Met Sci Heat Treat 26:476–482

Volynova TF, Emelyanova IZ, Sidorova IB (1992) Features of structure formation in Fe-Mn powder alloys during deformation and recrystallization. III. Effect of structure formation and recrystallization on alloy mechanical properties. Powder Metall Met Ceram 31:570–574

Xu WL, Lu X, Tan LL, Yang K (2011) Study on properties of a novel biodegradable Fe-30Mn-1C alloy. Acta Metall Sinica 47:1342–1347

Zvigintseva GY, Bogachev IN, Yegolayev VF (1970) Effect of carbon and silicon on the work hardening of the iron-manganese alloy G20. Phys Met Metallogr 30:61–67

Chapter 5
Metallic Biodegradable Coronary Stent: Degradation Study

Abstract Excellent mechanical properties and controllable degradation behavior without inducing toxicological problems are the key features of material for biodegradable stent. Iron-manganese alloys have shown comparable mechanical and physical properties to those of 316L stainless steel. Their degradation characteristics were then investigated including in vitro cell viability. A rather uniform corrosion mechanism was observed and metal hydroxides with calcium/phosphorus-containing layers were identified as degradation products. A low inhibition to fibroblast cells metabolic activities was noticed. The results demonstrated the potential of iron-manganese alloys to be developed as degradable metallic biomaterials.

Keywords Fe-Mn alloy · Biodegradable stent · Degradation · Cell viability

5.1 Static Degradation

Static degradation tests include potentiodynamic polarization and immersion method where the ASTM G59 and G31 standards (ASTM 2001a, b) can be viewed as a guidance. Degradation medium was prepared from Modified Hank's solution with HEPES buffer to maintain pH of the medium at 7.4 and its temperature was maintained at 37 ± 1 °C. Details on specimen preparation and test protocol can be found in Hermawan et al. (2010a).

Results from immersion tests showed no significant difference in degradation rate for all Fe-Mn alloys calculated from weight loss which was 0.23–0.24 mm/year. Similar rate was reported for pure Fe after immersion in Ringer solution which was 0.20–0.22 mm/year (Peuster et al. 2001). Table 5.1 presents degradation rate of Fe-Mn alloys calculated from weight loss and polarization measurement compared to pure Fe. Lower degradation rate by immersion could be due to

H. Hermawan, *Biodegradable Metals*, SpringerBriefs in Materials,
DOI: 10.1007/978-3-642-31170-3_5, © The Author(s) 2012

Table 5.1 Degradation rate of Fe-Mn alloys in comparison to pure Fe

Material	Degradation rate (mm/year)	
	Immersion	Potentiodynamic
Fe-20Mn	0.24 (0.04)	1.33 (0.07)
Fe-25Mn	0.24 (0.05)	1.08 (0.05)
Fe-30Mn	0.23 (0.05)	0.67 (0.06)
Fe-35Mn	0.23 (0.03)	0.44 (0.04)
Pure Fe[a]	0.20 (0.02)	0.16 (0.05)

Standard deviation is in parenthesis

[a] Pure Fe (99.8 % purity), annealed plate, Goodfellow Corporation, Oakdale, PA, USA

long immersion time (1 week), compared to short polarization time (15 min) that allowed the formation of degradation layer which inhibited further corrosion process.

The surface of specimens was covered by red-brownish hydroxide layer on the top and black-grayish oxide layer beneath. Four major elements in both layers: Fe, Mn, Cl and O were detected by energy dispersive spectrometer (EDS) whereas the first layer contained higher Fe and Cl but lower O than the second one. X-ray diffraction analysis revealed a typical non-crystalline spectrum but with some weak peaks corresponding to magnetite, Fe_3O_4 (JCPDS card no. 19-0629). Meanwhile, potentiodynamic polarization detected some differences where corrosion rate slightly increased as Mn content decreased.

5.2 Dynamic Degradation

Degradation tests were carried out in a test-bench that allow a laminar flow of testing solution to sweep specimens, which is similar to that published in Levesque et al. (2008). The Fe-25Mn and Fe-35Mn alloys which exhibit two different microstructures were chosen. Specimens with an exposed surface area of ~ 300 mm^2 were mounted in acrylic resin, polished using abrasive papers #1000, ultrasonically cleaned in 75 % ethanol, air-dried and stored 24 h in a desiccator prior to use. Degradation medium was prepared from Modified Hank's solution similar to that was used in Hermawan et al. (2010b).

A pseudo-physiological-like shear stress of 4 Pa was generated by a predetermined laminar flowing solution in the test bench, which is in the range of wall shear stress of human coronary arteries (Doriot et al. 2000). Details on the test bench, solution chemistry and test parameters are reported elsewhere (Levesque et al. 2008). The specimens were taken out after 1 week, 1 month and 3 months and were then characterized.

By measuring concentration of Fe and Mn in the degradation medium using atomic absorption spectrometer (AAS), an evolution of Fe and Mn ions release was approached and shown in Fig. 5.1.

Fig. 5.1 Concentration of Fe
and Mn ions in degradation
medium as a function of
immersion time for Fe-25Mn
and Fe-35Mn measured by
AAS. Adapted with
permission from Elsevier
(Hermawan et al. 2010b)

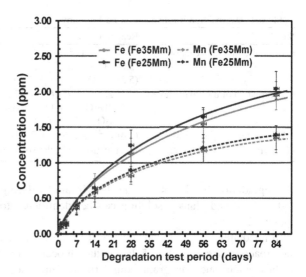

The curves indicate similarity in ion release for both alloys up to 14 days, but then Fe-25Mn released slightly more ions than Fe-35Mn. This measurement presented a complementary data on the rate of ions release. The highest average concentration reached after 3 months of degradation test was 2 ppm for Fe and 1.4 ppm for Mn in Fe-25Mn alloy. Those ion concentrations are very low compared to the experiment on AM60B Mg alloys that reached 50–100 ppm in 14 days (Levesque et al. 2008). This could be related to the fact that the degradation products of Fe-Mn alloys which contain Fe and Mn were not soluble.

The degradation product mostly adhered to the surface of specimens and was not completely washed out by the flowing solution, thus slowed down the ion exchange between the metal substrate and the solution. Characterization on degradation layer showed similar result as that of static degradation test. Further measurement by X-ray photoelectron spectrometer (XPS) revealed that the top layer contained mainly C, O, N, Na and trace of P, Cl and S. The presence of H could not be detected but it was expected as hydrated degradation products.

Degradation rate was also approached quantitatively by measuring the corroded depth as a function of degradation time. During the 3 months test period, the total corroded depth of Fe-25Mn specimens was 130 μm and that of Fe-35Mn specimens was 110 μm, corresponding to average degradation rates of 520 and 440 μm/year, respectively. The slightly faster degradation in Fe-25Mn could be related to the bi-phase composition where ε and γ phases coexist. Therefore, it presents more micro-galvanic sites susceptible to corrosion initiation than in Fe-35Mn which has only γ phase. Compared to pure Fe, which has corrosion rate of 220–240 μm/year (Peuster et al. 2001), both Fe-Mn alloys have shown higher corrosion rates. This could imply a faster in vivo degradation rate than pure Fe which was not completely degraded in rabbits after 18 months (Peuster et al. 2001). Meanwhile, the in vivo degradation is known to be much slower than that of in vitro (Witte et al. 2006).

Table 5.2 Degradation mechanism on Fe-Mn alloys

Step	Reaction
(1) Initial corrosion reaction	(5.1) $Fe \rightarrow Fe^{2+} + 2e^-$
	(5.2) $Mn \rightarrow Mn^{2+} + 2e^-$
	(5.3) $2H_2O + O_2 + 4e^- \rightarrow 4OH^-$
(2) Formation of hydroxide layers	(5.4) $2Fe^{2+} + 4OH^- \rightarrow 2Fe(OH)_2$ or $2FeO.2H_2O$
	(5.5) $4Fe(OH)_2 + O_2 + 2H_2O \rightarrow 4Fe(OH)_3$ or $2Fe_2O_3.$ $6H_2O$
(3) Formation of pits	(5.6) $Fe^{2+} + 2Cl^- \rightarrow FeCl_2 + H_2O \rightarrow Fe(OH)_2 + HCl$
(4) Formation of Ca/P layer	Precipitation from the solution

Degradation mechanism of the Fe-Mn alloys during the dynamic degradation test in modified Hank's solution can be identified into four steps as detailed in Table 5.2.

Immediately as the metal immersed in the degradation medium, initial corrosion reaction occurred, Fig. 5.2a. Oxidation occurred randomly at the more anodic surface spots such as grain boundaries or interface between different phases, Eqs. (5.1) and (5.2). A corresponding cathodic reaction (reduction of water) then consumed the released electrons, Eq. (5.3). Subsequently, insoluble hydroxides (hydrous metal oxides) layers were formed from the free metal ions that reacted with the hydroxyl ions (OH^-) following Eqs. (5.4) and (5.5), Fig. 5.2b. Under visual observation on the Fe-Mn specimens, those hydroxides appeared as red–brown (Fe_2O_3) layer on the top and black (Fe_3O_4 and FeO) layer on the bottom. Even though, XRD analysis rather detected only very weak peak pattern corresponds more to those of magnetite, Fe_3O_4. Based on literatures, degradation product of Fe alloys normally consisted of $FeO.nH_2O$ layer at the bottom, $Fe_3O_4.nH_2O$ in the middle and $Fe_2O_3.nH_2O$ on the top (Roberge 2000).

Chloride ions from the solution penetrated into metal substrate to compensate the increase of metal ions beneath the hydroxide layer. The formed metal chloride was then hydrolyzed into hydroxide and free acid, Eq. (5.6), lowering pH in the pits while the bulk solution remained neutral. Figure 5.2c illustrates this auto-catalytic reaction that lead to the formation and growth of pits (Shreir et al. 2000). As the degradation continued, a new Ca/P-contained-layer precipitated over the previously formed degradation layer, Fig. 5.2d.

5.3 In Vitro Cytotoxicity

Cell viability tests were carried out by indirect contact of metal samples with the 3T3 mouse fibroblast cell line by 3 μm tissue culture inserts. Powders of Fe-35Mn alloy, pure Fe, pure Mn and SS316L with average size less than 50 μm were used and their content in the medium was expressed as concentration (mg/ml). The water soluble tetrazolium (WST) assay was used to assess the cell viability after 48 h of incubation. Details on the protocol was published elsewhere (Hermawan et al. 2010b).

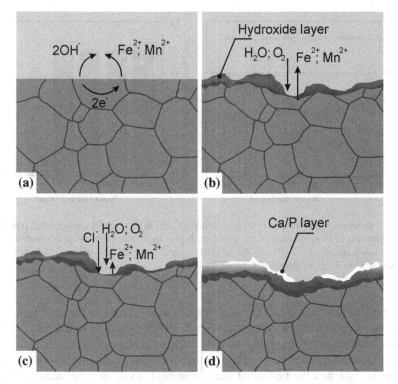

Fig. 5.2 Illustration for Fe-Mn alloys degradation mechanism: **a** initial reaction, **b** formation of hydroxide layer, **c** formation of pits, and **d** formation of Ca/P-contained layer. Adapted with permission from Elsevier (Hermawan et al. 2010b)

Figure 5.3a plots relative metabolic activity (RMA) of the 3T3 fibroblast cells to concentration of the metal samples. It indicates that Mn as the most toxic metal compared to Fe, SS316L and Fe-35Mn alloy. A sharp decline of RMA to less than 80 % was observed as the cells exposed to 0.01 mg/ml Mn powder, and was undetectable at 4 mg/ml. Contrary, the RMA of cells treated with Fe and SS316L remained as high as that of the control along the tested concentrations. Meanwhile, a distinct pattern was observed for Fe-35Mn sample where 0 % RMA was noted at 16 mg/ml or four times higher than that of Mn.

Further confirmation was done on fixed concentration of 0.5 mg/ml to show a good picture of inhibition. As shown in Fig. 5.3b, the RMA in presence of SS316L, Fe and Fe-35Mn alloy resembled to that of control. It was significantly higher than those of Mn and the mixture of Fe and Mn powders which add another evidence of low metabolic inhibition of Fe-35Mn alloy.

It is known that in most cases metal toxicity arises when reaction occurs between metals and body fluids acting as electrolytes. The metal ions that released during electrochemical reaction, e.g. Eqs. (5.1) and (5.2), are responsible for providing toxic effects (Flint 1998). However, it depends on the nature of the metal

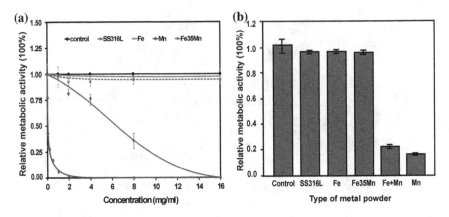

Fig. 5.3 Relative metabolic activity of 3T3 fibroblast cells in presence of various metal powders: **a** as a function of concentration of the powders, **b** at a fixed concentration of 0.5 mg/ml. *Note* Fe + Mn = mixture of 65wt% of Fe powder with 35wt% of Mn powder. Adapted with permission from Elsevier (Hermawan et al. 2010b)

ions itself against cell metabolic activities as clearly shown in Fig. 5.3. Iron is an essential element with a high toxic level, i.e. 350–500 µg/dl in serum (Frey 1999). Its low inhibition of metabolic activity can be explained by its characteristic where: (1) extracellular Fe bound to transferrin which maintains Fe soluble and non toxic, and then the Fe-loaded transferrin binds to its specific receptor on the cell surface and undergoes endocytosis; (2) the internalized excess of Fe is detoxified by sequestration into ferritin (Papanikolaou and Pantopoulos 2005). Meanwhile, SS316L is an inert metal where its low inhibition was mainly due to surface passivation of chromium oxide (Cr_2O_3) layer.

Manganese is also categorized as an essential element but with some toxic potential, i.e. a level of 3–5.6 µg/dl can cause neurologic symptoms (Ellenhorn et al. 1997). It may exist primarily in the form of Mn^{2+} (Harris and Chen 1994) but may be oxidized to a more reactive and more toxic Mn^{3+} (Chen et al. 2001). It targets mitochondria to cause high level of lactic acid (Hirata 2002) which then decrease the cells ability to cleave WST into soluble formazan, the parameter to measure cell viability. However, once Mn is alloyed with Fe to form a solid solution of metal alloy, the alloy's inhibition effect to the cell was reduced. The atoms in Fe-35Mn alloy arranged in a face centered cubic crystal structure known as the γ phase which is different than those of the forming elements, i.e. body centered cubic for Fe and simple cubic for Mn. Therefore, the alloy has very different characteristics than its forming elements. Figure 5.3 clearly shows that alloying significantly reduced the inhibition effect of Mn to the cells which is related to slow (small) release of Mn ion during dynamic degradation test (Fig. 5.1). If Fe and Mn powders were only mixed together without forming an alloy, the mixture, as shown in Fig. 5.3b, was still as toxic as Mn to the 3T3 fibroblast cells.

Table 5.3 Degradation and in vitro behavior of Fe-based biodegradable metals

Metal	Degradation rate (mm/year)	In vitro biological performance
Fe-Mn (Hermawan et al. 2010a)	0.44–1.33	Showed low inhibition to fibroblast cell viability
Fe electroformed (Moravej et al. 2010b)	0.46–1.22	Decreased proliferation of rat SMCs
Fe-30Mn-6Si (Liu et al. 2011)	0.30	Showed low hemolysis percentage (<2 %)
Fe-30Mn-1C (Xu et al. 2011)	0.14–0.22	Showed low hemolytic ratio and low platelet adhesion
Pure Fe (Moravej et al. 2010a)	0.16–0.19	Reduced growth rate of SMCs (Mueller et al. 2006)
Fe nanocrystalline (Nie et al. 2010)	0.09–0.20	Stimulated proliferation of fibroblast, promoted endothelialization and inhibited VSMCs viability
Fe-X (Liu and Zheng 2011)	0.10–0.17	Showed low hemolysis percentage (<5 %)

5.4 Conclusion and Benchmarking

Fe-Mn alloys degraded in vitro at an average rate up to 520 μm/year slightly faster than pure Fe with a mechanism rather uniform than localized. The degradation products constituted of iron hydroxides and calcium/phosphorus containing layers. The alloys possessed a low inhibition effect to 3T3 fibroblast cells metabolic activities compared to pure Mn. It can be concluded that Fe-Mn alloys have the potentiality to be a biocompatible degradable biomaterial with a degradation behavior considerably suitable for the development of stent.

Recent works on Fe-based alloys have shown improvement on mechanical property but not much improvement on degradation rate. The works also assessed more in vitro biological parameters to reveal the alloy's biocompatibility. Table 5.3 summarizes the degradation rate and some key in vitro biological performances of Fe-based biodegradable metals.

Xu et al. developed and compared Fe-30Mn and Fe-30Mn-1C alloys where the later showed a higher degradation rate than the earlier but still lower compared to Fe-30Mn developed by Hermawan et al. (Xu et al. 2011). Interestingly, Fe-30Mn-1C showed lower hemolytic ratio, better anticoagulation property and less platelet adhesion as well as good cell compatibility compared to Fe-30Mn which claimed as meeting the basic requirement on medical implants. Liu et al. have shown that corrosion rate of Fe-30Mn-6Si alloy was higher than that of Fe-30Mn alloy, beside also the alloy showed low hemolysis percentage (<2 %) which made it as a promising biodegradable metal with an interesting shape memory function (Liu et al. 2011).

The Fe-X (X = Mn, Co, Al, W, B, C or S) binary alloy models developed by Liu et al. showed degradation rates close to that of pure Fe which indicate no improvement compared to that of Fe-Mn alloys (Liu and Zheng 2011). The Fe-X binary alloys decreased the viability of the L929 cell line, maintained the viability of vascular smooth muscle cells (VSMCs) and increased the viability of the ECV304 cell line (except for Fe-Mn). All Fe-X binary alloy models resulted hemolysis percentage less than 5 % with no observed sign of thrombogenicity.

The degradation rate of pure Fe was not accelerated by changing its microstructure into nanocrystalline (Nie et al. 2010). However, the nanocrystalline pure Fe stimulated better proliferation of fibroblast cells and preferable promotion of endothelialization, while inhibits effectively the viability of VSMCs. In contact with the metal, the burst of red cells and adhesion of the platelets were also substantially suppressed in blood circulation. The work has shown that the refinement of microstructures correlated with well-behaved in vitro biocompatibility of Fe.

Differently, Moravej et al. have shown that pure Fe produced by electroforming degraded faster than conventional cast pure Fe (Moravej et al. 2010b). The metal did not decrease the metabolic activity of primary rat smooth muscle cells but it decreased the cell proliferation activity which could be beneficial for the inhibition of in-stent restenosis.

References

ASTM (2001a) ASTM G 31: standard practice for laboratory immersion corrosion testing of metals. ASTM International, West Conshohocken

ASTM (2001b) ASTM G 59: standard test method for conducting potentiodynamic polarization resistance measurements. ASTM International, West Conshohocken

Chen JY, Tsao GC, Zhao Q, Zheng W (2001) Differential cytotoxicity of Mn(II) and Mn(III): special reference to mitochondrial [Fe–S] containing enzymes. Toxicol Appl Pharmacol 175:160–168

Doriot PA, Dorsaz PA, Dorsaz L, De Benedetti E, Chatelain P, Delafontaine P (2000) In vivo measurements of wall shear stress in human coronary arteries. Coron Artery Dis 11:495–502

Ellenhorn MJ, Schonwald S, Ordog G, Wasserberger J (1997) Ellenhorn's medical toxicology: diagnosis and treatment of human poisoning. Williams & Wilkins, Baltimore

Flint GN (1998) A metallurgical approach to metal contact dermatitis. Cont Dermat 39:213–221

Frey RJ (1999) Iron tests. In: Gale encyclopaedia of medicine. Gale Research, Detroit

Harris RW, Chen Y (1994) Electron paramagnetic resonance and difference ultraviolet studies of Mn2+ binding to serum transferrin. J Inorg Biochem 54:1–19

Hermawan H, Dube D, Mantovani D (2010a) Degradable metallic biomaterials: design and development of Fe-Mn alloys for stents. J Biomed Mater Res A 93:11

Hermawan H, Purnama A, Dube D, Couet J, Mantovani D (2010b) Fe-Mn alloys for metallic biodegradable stents: degradation and cell viability studies. Acta Biomater 6:1852–1860

Hirata Y (2002) Manganese-induced apoptosis in PC12 cells. Neurotoxicol Teratol 24:639–653

Levesque J, Hermawan H, Dube D, Mantovani D (2008) Design of a pseudo-physiological test bench specific to the development of biodegradable metallic biomaterials. Acta Biomater 4:284–295

Liu B, Zheng YF (2011) Effects of alloying elements (Mn, Co., Al, W, Sn, B, C and S) on biodegradability and in vitro biocompatibility of pure iron. Acta Biomater 7:1407–1420

Liu B, Zheng YF, Ruan L (2011) In vitro investigation of Fe30Mn6Si shape memory alloy as potential biodegradable metallic material. Mater Lett 65:540–543

Moravej M, Prima F, Fiset M, Mantovani D (2010a) Electroformed iron as new biomaterial for degradable stents: development process and structure-properties relationship. Acta Biomater 6:1726–1735

Moravej M, Purnama A, Fiset M, Couet J, Mantovani D (2010b) Electroformed iron as new biomaterial for degradable stents: in vitro degradation and preliminary cell viability studies. Acta Biomater 6:1843–1851

Mueller PP, May T, Perz A, Hauser H, Peuster M (2006) Control of smooth muscle cell proliferation by ferrous iron. Biomaterials 27(10):2193–2200

Nie FL, Zheng YF, Wei SC, Hu C, Yang G (2010) In vitro corrosion, cytotoxicity and hemocompatibility of bulk nanocrystalline pure iron. Biomed Mater 5:065015

Papanikolaou G, Pantopoulos K (2005) Iron metabolism and toxicity. Toxicol Appl Pharmacol 202:199–211

Peuster M, Wohlsein P, Brugmann M, Ehlerding M, Seidler K, Fink C, Brauer H, Fischer A, Hausdorf G (2001) A novel approach to temporary stenting: degradable cardiovascular stents produced from corrodible metal-results 6–18 months after implantation into New Zealand white rabbits. Heart 86:563–569

Roberge PR (2000) Handbook of corrosion engineering. McGraw-Hill, Toronto

Shreir LL, Jarman RA, Burstein GT (2000) Corrosion, metal/environment reactions, vol 1, 3rd edn. Butterworth-Heinemann, Oxford

Witte F, Fischer J, Nellesen J, Crostack H-A, Kaese V, Pisch A, Beckmann F, Windhagen H (2006) In vitro and in vivo corrosion measurements of magnesium alloys. Biomaterials 27:1013–1018

Xu WL, Lu X, Tan LL, Yang K (2011) Study on properties of a novel biodegradable Fe-30Mn-1C alloy. Acta Metall Sinica 47:1342–1347

Chapter 6
Metallic Biodegradable Coronary Stent: Stent Prototyping

Abstract Iron-manganese alloys have been designed, developed and assessed as material for biodegradable metallic coronary stent. The alloys have shown mechanical and physical properties comparable to those of 316L stainless steel and suitable in vitro degradation behavior. Therefore, it is interesting to transform the alloys into stent prototype, to determine their processability and to assess the implant properties. The current available technology of stent processing might be adapted to fabricate biodegradable stents. This chapter covers fabrication of iron-manganese stents that followed a standard process for fabricating and testing 316L stainless steel stents. It was found that some steps like laser cutting can be directly applied; but changes on the parameters are needed for annealing and alternatives are needed to replace electropolishing.

Keywords Biodegradable stent · Stent fabrication · Laser cutting · Annealing · Descaling · Fe-Mn alloy

6.1 Stent Design

The Fe-35Mn alloy was selected as material for fabrication of Fe-Mn stent prototypes. It was produced from elemental powders of high purity Fe and Mn through powder sintering and thermo-mechanical treatments as detailed in the previous chapter as well as in (Hermawan et al. 2008). The alloy composed of 35.3wt% Mn, 0.04wt% C, 0.006wt% Si, 0.0224wt% O, 0.005wt% N and balanced with Fe. Its mechanical property is detailed in Table 6.1.

An industrial protocol for fabricating SS316L stents involving laser cutting, annealing, descaling and electropolishing, as reviewed in (Hermawan et al. 2010a), was followed. Standard characterization methods as for SS316L stents was applied to the developed stent prototypes. A structure of a commercial SS316L stent was

Table 6.1 Mechanical properties of the Fe-35Mn alloy and SS316L

Material	Tensile strength (MPa)	Yield strength (MPa)	Maximum elongation (%)
Fe-35Mn	550 ± 8	235 ± 8	31 ± 5
SS316L	580 ± 2	250 ± 2	56 ± 2

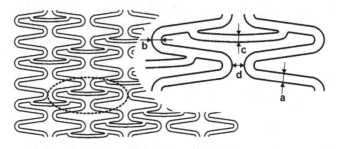

Fig. 6.1 2-D projection of designed stent and important strut measurement (*inset*), *a* strut, *b* curvature, *c* connector, *d* width between curves

redrawn by using a computer aided design (CAD) program and was taken as the model for the developed stent as shown in Fig. 6.1.

6.2 Minitube Fabrication

Tube extrusion or cold drawing is a common method for mass producing SS316L minitubes for stents as they provide excellent dimensional accuracy and induce cold-worked condition for the ease of handling and fixturing (Poncin and Proft 2003). Extrusion was also used in producing minitubes for the experimental Mg-based alloys stents (Hassel et al. 2007). However, for Fe-35Mn stent prototyping, the minitube was made by means of machining process (Fig. 6.2). The bulk material was machined into rectangular bars by using electrical discharge wire cutter, and then into minitubes by employing high precision drilling and turning machineries. The micro dimension of the minitubes, 1.80 mm (±0.01) of outside diameter, 0.15 mm (±0.0075) of wall thickness, and 40 mm of length, was achieved without any major problem in fixturing or bending.

6.3 Stent Fabrication

6.3.1 Laser Cutting

The Fe-35Mn minitubes were cut following the programmed stent design by means of an Nd-YAG laser cutting machine with oxygen as cutting gas (Rofin-Baasel

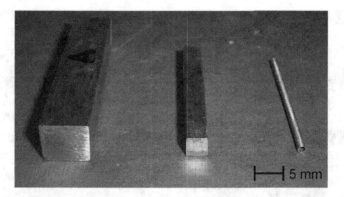

Fig. 6.2 Transformation of Fe-35Mn alloy from bulk material made though PM machined into minitube

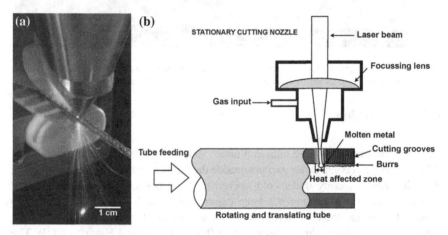

Fig. 6.3 Laser cutting process of stents: **a** photograph, **b** schematic illustration. Adapted with permission from Bentham Science (Hermawan et al. 2010b)

Lasertech, Starnberg, Germany). The cutting parameters were set at: wavelength = 1064 nm, pulse frequency = 5300 Hz, pulse duration/pulse width = 10 μs and nominal power = 100 W. Figure 6.3 shows a typical laser cutting process for stents, meanwhile the transformation of a Fe-35Mn minitube into stent is shown by scanning electron microscope (SEM) images in Fig. 6.4. The minitube was successfully laser cut using the same parameters as for SS316L stents (Figs. 6.4a, b).

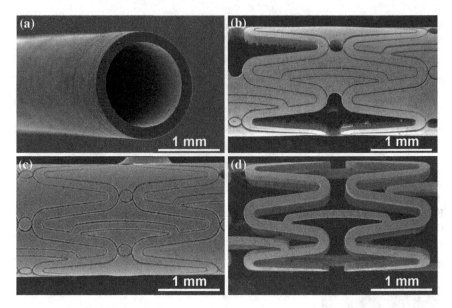

Fig. 6.4 SEM images on the evolution from minitube to stent: **a** initial machined minitube, **b** laser cut minitube, **c** annealed laser cut minitube, and **d** descaled minitube (stent)

6.3.2 Annealing

The laser cut minitubes were annealed under 100 Pa vacuum pressure at 900 °C for 20 min, and then cooled under vacuum outside the furnace. In SS316L stent fabrication, the minitubes is usually under cold-worked to avoid bending and scratches during handling, therefore annealing has been commonly applied. It brings the stent into annealed condition thereby increase ductility and eliminate possible microstructural inhomogeneity induced during laser cutting (Meyer-Kobbe and Hinrichs 2003). The later was also expected for Fe-35Mn stent. Figure 6.4c shows the laser cut minitube after annealing.

6.3.3 Descaling

This term was used to name the process to remove non-stent parts from the annealed laser cut minitubes. Acid pickling is another term often used for SS316L stents. Different with that for SS316L, descaling parameters applied for Fe-35Mn were: (1) immersion in acidic solution composed of 5 % H_3PO_4 + 0.5 % H_2O_2 + water at 60 °C for 30–60 s under ultrasonic vibration, (2) rinsing in deionised water and then ethanol all under ultrasonic vibration and dried in open air. After descaling, burrs (remelted material on minitube's inner surfaces) and slags (remelted material on cutting walls) attached to the cutting line were

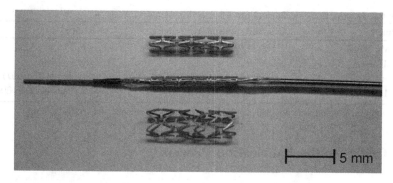

Fig. 6.5 Photograph of Fe-35Mn stents at three conditions: (*up*) as descaled, (*middle*) as crimped over balloon, and (*bottom*) as expanded

dissolved allowing the non-stent parts to be successfully removed and to easily recover the stent. The weight of descaled stents was ~15 mg each.

6.4 Stent's Mechanical Testing

Expansion test was done following the same protocol as applied for SS316L stents as shown in Fig. 6.5.

The Fe-35Mn stents were crimped over balloon catheter using a manual crimper where stent's diameter shrunk from 1.80 to 1.05 mm. The catheter was then connected with a manual pump which delivered water to gradually inflate the balloon up to its maximum diameter of 3.0 mm (French scale 9). The stents were fully expanded at 6 atm. The expanded diameter of stents while still on the inflated balloon was 3.15 mm and shrunk (recoiled) to 3.10 when the pressure was released. The un-cracked or un-ruptured stents observed under stereo microscope were then sent for mechanical tests.

Results from mechanical tests (Table 6.2) showed that Fe-35Mn stent possessed lower radial force but similar recoil compared to the similarly designed SS316L stents. However, compared to other metallic biodegradable stents, Fe-35Mn stent has higher radial force than Biotronik absorbable Mg stent (AMS), and lower recoil than both AMS and NOR-1 Fe stent.

Mechanical property of the Fe-35Mn stents can be further improved by optimizing the physical and metallurgical aspects of the stents. Better expansion behavior, i.e. less crack or strut rupture is expected when smoother surface can be obtained. Higher radial force is also expected once the metallurgical condition of the stents can be improved, i.e. number of grains across the strut thickness higher than ten.

Table 6.2 Results from mechanical test of Fe-35Mn stents

Specimen	Radial force (mN)	Recoil (%)
Fe-35Mn stents	1800 ± 200	<1
SS316L stents	3800 ± 50	<1
Biotronik AMS	~800 (Zartner et al. 2005)	8 (Erbel et al. 2007)
NOR-1 Fe stent	N/A	2.2 (Peuster et al. 2006)

Note Different method was possibly applied to test AMS Biotronik and NOR-1 stents

6.5 Critics to the Fabrication Process

Annealing should not be carried out under vacuum. Alternatively, annealing under argon at pressure higher than vapor pressure of Mn or annealing under Mn-rich inert atmosphere could be a suitable process. For the used Fe-Mn alloy, annealing after laser cutting might not be necessary since the initial minitube condition was already annealed and since the laser cutting did not induce any substantial microstructural change.

Minitubes fabrication by machining limits the length of the tubes since it depend on the length and rigidity of the drilling bit/rod. Tube drawing or extrusion should be more suitable as it is commonly employed for making long, consistent and dimensional accurate SS316L minitubes for stents.

Electropolishing as the common process for improving surface condition of SS316L stents might not be suitable for metallic biodegradable stents since the use of acidic solution in conjunction with electrical current causes relatively uncontrolled corrosion attacks on relatively non-uniform surface condition of the stents after descaling. Microblasting could be a potential alternative to be performed after descaling to improve surface condition of metallic biodegradable stents. The impingement of micro-balls will theoretically reduce surface roughness and close surface porosity. In addition, blasting could also introduce superficial compressive residual stress which is beneficial to prevent crack initiation and propagation.

6.6 Stent's Degradation Testing

A stent is inserted into a narrowed coronary artery by using a catheter system through a small incision in arm or groin (King et al. 2008). The whole procedure may take 1.5–2.5 h (Texas Heart Insitute 2010), but the time frame for a stent starting from insertion until deployment may take about 15 to 30 min. During that time frame the stent was always in contact with blood, a corrosive and warm environment. For a biodegradable stent, degradation process should already begin in that time. Therefore, an observation to stent degradation during its early period of implantation was conducted.

The degradation test was carried out in a test-bench that simulated conditions in human coronary arteries as detailed in (Levesque et al. 2008). Testing solution was

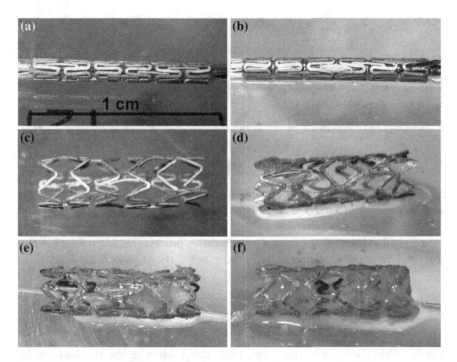

Fig. 6.6 Photographs of the Fe-35Mn stents: **a, b** crimped, before and after 0.5 h of degradation test, **c, d, e, f** expanded before and after degradation test: 1, 24, a week, respectively

prepared from Modified Hank's solution which was circulated at velocity of 10 cm/s to create a laminar flow inside the test channel. The flow introduced a calculated shear stress on the stents as 0.6 Pa which was in the range of wall shear stress of human coronary arteries (Doriot et al. 2000). Figure 6.6 shows photographs of stent specimens before and after degradation tests taken immediately after they were taken-off from the test-bench.

The stents can be stably crimped without problem of non-uniformity or displacement (Fig. 6.6a) and be fully expanded (Fig. 6.6c) without rupture. Only the stents, which visually (40X magnification) have no fissure or crack after expansion, were then used for degradation tests. Figure 6.6b shows that there was no sign of visible corrosion attack on crimped stent after 0.5 h of degradation test. Meanwhile, a progression of corrosion was well visible on expanded stents as degradation period extended (Figs. 6.6d, e, f) as shown by the change of color and formation of corrosion product.

Figure 6.7 shows SEM images of the surface of the stent after 24 h of degradation test where by using EDS these elements were detected: 55wt% Fe, 7wt% Mn, 5wt% P, 3wt% Ca, 4wt% Na and 26wt% O. It was also detected that precipitation of Ca and P on crimped stent as early as 0.5 h of degradation test. As the test period extended, the amount of P, Ca, Na and O increased but the amount of Fe and Mn decreased. This could be due to the formation of oxide layer

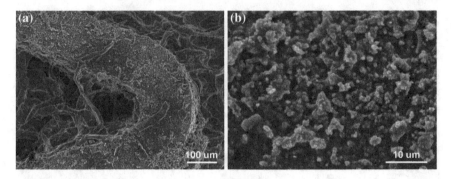

Fig. 6.7 Surface morphology of the Fe-35Mn stents after 24 h of degradation test: **a** a curvature, and **b** magnification of a region on **a**

(+precipitation layer) slows down the degradation process (Fe, Mn release) as also described during degradation study of the material (Hermawan et al. 2010b).

6.7 Conclusion

The Fe-35Mn alloy can be transformed into stents following the standard process for SS316L stents with some modifications on the processing parameters. The produced Fe-35Mn stents shows an acceptable overall mechanical property. Physical aspects of the stent can be considered unacceptable for their excessive surface roughness. Further improvement to some process parameters and finding new alternative additional process are mandatory. Modification to metallurgical condition of the alloy is also necessary. The Fe-35Mn stent starts to degrade as soon as it is intact with degradation medium. The stents maintain its mechanical integrity during a short-term degradation test up to 1 week.

6.8 Suggestion

Beside mechanical and long-term degradation tests, a short-term degradation test protocol on biodegradable stents could be mandatory. This test is to confirm that on the very early period, from stent insertion into arterial system till expansion, the stents is not severely degraded which can cause rupture during expansion. This confirmation will ensure that the deployed stent has a perfect integrity to fulfill its function and to degrade away as expected.

The test should involve two situations: (1) immersion of a crimped stent over balloon catheter in a flowing SBF for a short period, i.e. 30 min; and (2) expansion of the stent in the flowing SBF. The expanded stent is then observed under microscope with sufficient magnification for any sign of crack or rupture.

References

Doriot PA, Dorsaz PA, Dorsaz L, De Benedetti E, Chatelain P, Delafontaine P (2000) In vivo measurements of wall shear stress in human coronary arteries. Coron Artery Dis 11:495–502

Erbel R, Di Mario C, Bartunek J, Bonnier J, de Bruyne B, Eberli FR, Erne P, Haude M, Heublein B, Horrigan M, Ilsley C, Bose D, Koolen J, Luscher TF, Weissman N, Waksman R (2007) Temporary scaffolding of coronary arteries with bioabsorbable magnesium stents: a prospective, non-randomised multicentre trial. Lancet 369:1869–1875

Hassel T, Bach F-W, Golovko AN (2007) Production and properties of small tubes made from MgCa0.8 for application as stent in biomedical science. In: Kainer KU (ed) Proceedings of 7th international conference on magnesium alloys and their applications, Dresden

Hermawan H, Alamdari H, Mantovani D, Dubé D (2008) Iron-manganese: new class of degradable metallic biomaterials prepared by powder metallurgy. Powder Metall 51:38–45

Hermawan H, Dubé D, Mantovani D (2010a) Patents on metallic biodegradable stents. Rec Patent Mater Sci 3:140–145

Hermawan H, Purnama A, Dube D, Couet J, Mantovani D (2010b) Fe-Mn alloys for metallic biodegradable stents: degradation and cell viability studies. Acta Biomater 6:1852–1860

Texas Heart Insitute (2010) Balloon angioplasty and stents. http://www.texasheartinstitute.org/HIC/Topics/Proced/angioplasty.cfm. Accessed 15 Apr 2010

King SB, Hirshfeld JW, Williams DO, Feldman TE, Kern MJ, O'Neill WW, Williams DO, Jacobs AK, Buller CE, Hunt SA, Lytle BW, Tarkington LG, Yancy CW (2008) 2007 focused update of the ACC/AHA/SCAI 2005 guideline update for percutaneous coronary intervention. Circulation 117:261–295

Levesque J, Hermawan H, Dube D, Mantovani D (2008) Design of a pseudo-physiological test bench specific to the development of biodegradable metallic biomaterials. Acta Biomater 4:284–295

Meyer-Kobbe C, Hinrichs BH (2003) The importance of annealing 316 LVM stent. Med Device Technol 14:20–25

Peuster M, Beerbaum P, Bach FW, Hauser H (2006) Are resorbable implants about to become a reality? Cardiol Young 16:107–116

Poncin P, Proft J (2003) Stent tubing: understanding the desired attributes. In: Materials & processes for medical devices conference, California, 8–10 September 2003, ASM International

Zartner P, Cesnjevar R, Singer H, Weyand M (2005) First successful implantation of a biodegradable metal stent into the left pulmonary artery of a preterm baby. Catheter Cardiovasc Interv 66:590–594

Chapter 7
Perspective

The advance in tissue engineering has demanded biomaterials to exhibit bio-functional capability. The future direction for metallic implants goes toward the combination of the superior mechanical property of metals and the excellent bio-functionality of ceramics and polymers. A future for metallic biomaterials may include their revolutionary use for biodegradable implants. The study of innovative biodegradable metals is one of the most interesting research topics at the forefront of biomaterials in present days.

Introduced in 2001 when pure iron was used to make stent prototype and tested in rabbits, biodegradable metals have attracted interest of biomaterialists. Hundred studies have been published till the most significant clinical study of absorbable magnesium stents for treatment of critical limb ischemia in 2009. However, a significant breakthrough has never been reported. It has been ten years of development but there is still lack of knowledge which prevented the clinical use of this emerging technology.

There are at least two questions remain unexplained very well in biodegradable metals, namely: (1) the interaction between metal and its degradation product with the surrounding implantation site, and (2) in vivo degradation mechanism and its kinetics.

Very recently, a workshop on the state of the art of biodegradable metals was held in the FDA's Silver Spring office on 30th March 2012 attended by 120 participants. The aim of the workshop was to bring the current knowledge in this field and to discuss the current view of the FDA on this emerging technology. The workshop came out with an initiative to form a standardization committee on biodegradable metals for medical use. This may indicate a future for the applications of biodegradable metals in the medical field.

H. Hermawan, *Biodegradable Metals*, SpringerBriefs in Materials, DOI: 10.1007/978-3-642-31170-3_7, © The Author(s) 2012